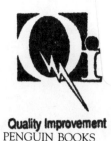

Quality Improvement
PENGUIN BOOKS

VICTORIA JOHNSON'S ATTITUDE

Victoria Johnson lives in Portland, Oregon, and stands as one of the most influential professionals in the aerobics industry today. A seventeen-year aerobic and dance veteran, Ms. Johnson is the creator of her own international workout video series. Her work has also been praised in national publications such as *USA Today*, *Self*, *Shape*, *Essence*, *Black Enterprise*, and *Vogue*. Technifunk™ 2000, Ms. Johnson's dance workout video, won the distinction Funk Video of the Year from *Self*, *American Health*, and *American Fitness* magazines. Dubbed the "Michael Jordan of aerobics" by executives at L.A. Gear, Ms. Johnson is a fitness trendsetter who now reigns as the Dance Diva and spokeswoman for L.A. Gear. Ms. Johnson is also a certified instructor and continuing-education provider for ACE (American Council on Exercise) and AFAA (Aerobics and Fitness Association of America) and travels the world educating other instructors on the latest industry information.

Megan V. Davis was born in Michigan in 1959, and received her bachelor of arts degree in English literature from the University of Michigan in 1981. A former elementary/high school textbook sales representative for West Publishing Company, she began her free-lance writing career in the mid-1980s. Ms. Davis lives in Portland, Oregon, with her husband, Don, and her two children, Alison and Kendall. *Victoria Johnson's Attitude* is her first book.

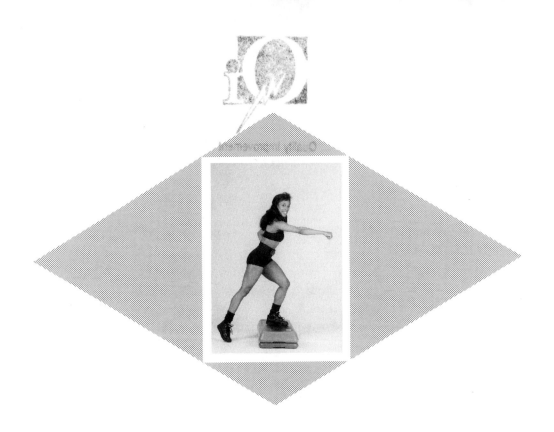

VICTORIA JOHNSON

WITH MEGAN V. DAVIS

Penguin Books

Victoria Johnson's

◀ ATTITUDE ▶

AN

INSPIRATIONAL GUIDE

TO REDEFINING

YOUR BODY, YOUR HEALTH,

AND YOUR OUTLOOK

PENGUIN BOOKS
Published by the Penguin Group
Viking Penguin, a division of Penguin Books USA Inc.,
375 Hudson Street, New York, New York 10014, U.S.A.
Penguin Books Ltd, 27 Wrights Lane, London W8 5TZ, England
Penguin Books Australia Ltd, Ringwood, Victoria, Australia
Penguin Books Canada Ltd, 10 Alcorn Avenue, Suite 300, Toronto, Ontario, Canada M4V 3B2
Penguin Books (N.Z.) Ltd, 182–190 Wairau Road, Auckland 10, New Zealand

Penguin Books Ltd, Registered Offices:
Harmondsworth, Middlesex, England

First published in Penguin Books 1993

1   3   5   7   9   10   8   6   4   2

Photographs: Sam Potts

LIBRARY OF CONGRESS CATALOGING IN PUBLICATION DATA
Johnson, Victoria.
Victoria Johnson's attitude : an inspirational guide to redefining
your body, your health, and your outlook / Victoria Johnson with
Megan V. Davis.
p.   cm.
ISBN 0 14 01.7537 7
1. Aerobic exercises.   2. Aerobic exercises—Psychological
aspects.   3. Physical fitness.   4. Mind and body.   I. Davis, Megan V.
II. Title.
RA781.15.J65   1993
613.7′1—dc20   92–23360

Printed in the United States of America
Set in Goudy Old Style
Designed by Claire Vaccaro

I would like to dedicate this book to my grandmother:

Pearl Ann Dimmer
1906–1991

Pearl taught me that learning was a privilege.
She taught me that color
was not a barrier. Most of all she taught me
that giving was by far greater
than receiving.

—Victoria Johnson

For my parents, Curt and Beth Van Voorhees—
the loudest voices in my cheering section.
With love.

—Megan V. Davis

Dear Victoria:
Your classes have saved my soul!
You've helped me move
forward toward my goals
When things were bad and
life didn't seem worth it
Taking your classes always
gave me rebirth—
it seems such a small thing—
music and motion
But I give you my thanks
with heartfelt emotion!

Written to Victoria by one of her students

Foreword

Rap music blasts through two wide-open doors, its beat pounding and rhythmic. Inside the room, thirty sweat-covered bodies move in complete unison. All eyes are riveted on the front of the room, fixed on a small, muscular woman decked out in cotton and Lycra spandex. With one hand twisting in the air and the other wrapped around a microphone, the woman smiles, kicks, and makes jokes. In a sudden blur of movement, she leaps from her position to weave among the crowd.

"All right, now, this time concentrate on your technique. Lift that leg and squeeze those buns. Come on, you can do it. Remember, if you don't squeeze them . . ." The class responds on cue, ". . . nobody else will."

Anyone who thinks there is no such thing as a perpetual-motion machine has not met Victoria Johnson. Just to take one of her aerobics classes is to experience nonstop energy and enthusiasm.

"Count with me now . . . three, two, one. Oh, sweatin' a little bit there—huh, Joe? Yeah! We *love* to sweat! You guys look great! Nice job! I love your *attitudes!*"

Can you believe this is a woman who once tipped the scales at 175 pounds?

Can you believe this is a woman once paralyzed with fear when speaking in front of a crowd?

Can you believe this is a woman who could devour half a gallon of ice cream and an entire chocolate cake in one sitting?

Believe it! This woman is in all of us, and her ability to change is within us as well.

Victoria Johnson has "attitude" written all over her. She symbolizes how adversity can be converted into personal power and success. Her story is one of suffering and self-destruction, but ultimately one of revelation and transformation. The bottom line of Victoria's message is one of care and concern: "People know I am real, I am authentic, I have been there. And yes, it is possible to pull yourself up; you *can* succeed." Let her show you how.

—M. V. D.

Acknowledgments

VICTORIA JOHNSON:

I would like to thank all my many friends and the thousands of students who have let me teach and share my passion for aerobics over the past seventeen years. Thank you to my chiropractor and friend, Dr. Mark Butterfield, for keeping my body healthy through the years. Thank you to my special true friends who have been there, nurtured me, and believed in my dreams: Jimi, Artie, Billie, and Sally.

I would also like to thank the hardworking team who made this entire project physically possible. Thank you, Megan Davis, a very special lady, my writer who now has *soul!* Thank you, Jennifer Lauck, my publicist, friend, and the most awesome Step & Funk instructor in town.

Thanks to my mother, Pankie Lee, and my father, Ernest, for teaching me that there are no mountains too high to climb, and for teaching me that if you want it, you can get it; you just have to earn it!

And, thanks to my dear and loving family—Daniel, Cecily, Jesse, and David.

MEGAN V. DAVIS:

There were many special people who shared in the development of this book. First, my heartfelt thanks to my agent, Linda Chester, and to her assistant, Laurie Fox, for their belief in this project from its earliest phases and for their persistence in finding it a home. Second, my thanks to my husband, Don, for his nonstop encouragement and support throughout my various moods and periods of self-doubt. Third, I thank my children, Alison and Kendall, who showed remarkable patience even after Mommy promised "Just one more page" and then kept right on typing. Fourth, many thanks to all my kind friends who cared for my children so that I could work without interruptions (I *owe* you!). Fifth, thank you to Jennifer Lauck at Metro Fitness, Inc., for her invaluable assistance over the past year and a half. And finally, to Vic: Thank you for letting me share the Attitude—we did it, *girlfriend!*

Contents

Introduction

Attitude!

Remember when "attitude" was something your parents wanted you to change? Did your mother or father ever say something like, "You'd better change your attitude right now and go clean up that room of yours," or "Young lady, I don't like your attitude"? Having an "attitude" got you into trouble—you forfeited your allowance because of it or you got grounded, and you probably drove your poor parents crazy.

Today, "attitude" has taken on a new meaning. While it's true that someone can still have a *bad* attitude or an attitude *problem*, for the most part the word has shed its negative image and become an accepted term for high self-esteem and self-confidence. Sometimes when I'm teaching aerobics I'll call out to the class, "Show me some attitude!" Obviously, I'm not telling my students to snatch up their towels and stomp off to the locker room in a huff—just the opposite. I'm telling them to hold their heads up high, to straighten up their shoulders and show me they're proud of who they are. I want them to have fun and to love life; after all, *life* is not a rehearsal. For me, "attitude" is a philosophy—one that emphasizes personal strength and style, self-empowerment, confidence, energy, and enthusiasm—and

▼

You have to feel good to look good.

xiii

it's at the core of my message about mental well-being and physical fitness.

In general, I think we all tend to focus too much on the negatives in our lives. Without doubt, it's difficult not to be angered and upset by many of the happenings around us. And as if such external events weren't enough to cast us into a permanent state of gloom and doom, the internal "tapes" that each of us listens to on a daily basis also play us the following messages: You're not good enough, you're too fat, you never do anything right, you're a terrible parent, you're a lousy partner, you always say the wrong thing, you'll never succeed at anything, and on, and on, and on. If they are played too often and too loudly, eventually we start believing those tapes and living our lives as if the tapes actually had some basis in reality; they exit our subconscious mind and dictate our conscious existence.

Victoria Johnson's Attitude is about pushing the "eject" button and getting rid of those negative, self-defeating tapes running through your head. This book is about positive thinking and taking positive action, believing in yourself and taking control of your life. It's about valuing your health and making a commitment to improve your level of physical fitness. It's about *motion creating emotion*. When you're moving, you become more alert and excited—more oxygen goes throughout your body, your eyes have more sparkle. It's hard to be depressed when you're moving quickly, dancing to high-energy music and smiling.

I care enough to want to improve the quality of your life—that's why I'm in this fitness business, and that's why I wrote this book. I want to inspire you to *take action* and assist you in changing your life; I want to make you a happier, healthier, more effective human being. In short, I want to teach you how to get an "attitude." But in order for you to let me do that, first you need to understand and trust me. You need to see where I've been . . .

▼

What you think is what you are.

▼

Without the physical energy it's difficult to have the mental energy.

▼

People don't care how much you know, until they know how much you care.

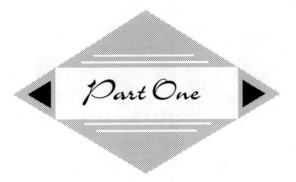

Part One

OUR
OWN STORIES
TO TELL

It's not what happens to you in life; it's how you
think about what happens that really matters.

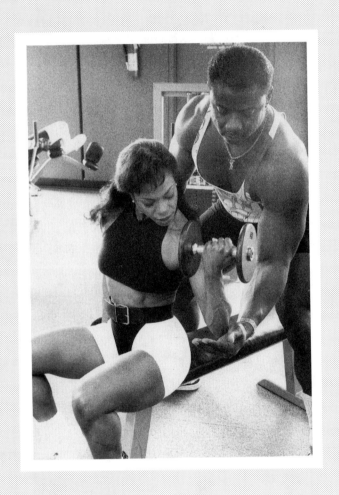

Chapter One:
My Story

A Diet Diva

For almost two decades I was the Queen of Dieting. From the "Egg and Spinach Diet" to the "Grapefruit 45 Plan (Lose 45 Pounds in 45 Days!)" to the "Burn Fat While You Sleep Diet," I tried them all. On a never-ending quest for the "miracle quick-fix reduction plan," I watched my weight bounce back and forth like a yo-yo for twenty years: overweight, underweight, up, down, up, down. Little did I know how destructive this pattern was. Not only did my body pay a high price for my excessive dieting, but the effects on my psyche were devastating, too. Here's how it all began . . .

Born in Louisiana, I was number six in a family of eleven children. My father and mother harvested fruit and vegetables for a living. When I was three, we moved west to Yakima Valley, a migrant community in central Washington. For years we traveled back and forth, from the south to the west, following the crop cycles. We spent summer and fall in Washington for the fruit harvests; in winter and spring we returned to Louisiana because of school and to visit our relatives. The houses that my father could afford to rent had dirt floors and tiny rooms, but if we had a roof over our heads and food on the table, we felt we were doing all right. We took each day as it came.

The concept of preparing for the future—of having goals and saving money—was something we never discussed. Survival on a daily basis was our primary agenda.

As far back as I can remember, mealtimes were the highlight of our days. For me, mealtimes were the only times I felt we were a "normal" family, not some migrant family who barely made ends meet. How could we be *poor*, after all, when there was so much food on the table? Mealtimes were also the main source of family entertainment and a welcome relief from the harsh and sometimes frightening realities of life in a migrant community. After everyone's chores were finished at the end of the day, we all sat crowded around the table eating, laughing, joking, and listening to the wonderful stories my father told about his childhood. Desperately wanting to prolong these happy moments, I'd reload my supper plate and beg my father to continue long after the others had left the table. Eventually, food came to symbolize a means of escape for me. Food comforted my soul and made me forget, at least for a while, the difficult life we led.

I was already overweight by the age of five, and it's no wonder! Not only did I have a large appetite, but the foods I ate were high in fat and low on the nutritional scale: biscuits, ham, eggs, fried chicken, cakes, butter, cream, and gravy galore. At five years old, my looks didn't concern me a whole lot; I was the same as everyone else around me, and that's what mattered most.

As children we were expected to work alongside our parents in the fields. I can still picture my mother, her belly bulging with another child, high atop a ladder picking apples or hunched over all day picking asparagus. She'd work right up to the baby's birth and two weeks later be back in the fields again. My brothers, sisters, and I were up at four in the morning to help with the crops before school. We worked after school, in the evenings, and all summer long. Sometimes we had to stay home from school to work in the fields. If government truant officers drove up in their big white cars, we'd dart up the fruit trees or scramble under our beds so we wouldn't get caught.

Still, education was important to my parents. Their search for racial equality and a better education for their children was what had brought us west initially, and eventually we stayed in Washington. My grandmother taught me that learning was a privilege, not a given. And she knew what she was talking about; her mother had been a slave and had not been allowed to read. My grandmother taught me that reading was the avenue to power and control, and that if I ever wanted to get ahead in life I'd better learn to read and study hard. She also taught me it's not what happens to you in life, it's how you *think* about what happens that really matters. Having experienced more than her own share of heartaches in her lifetime, my grandmother was a constant source of inspiration and an important influence on me as I grew up.

When I entered first grade, my perception of myself changed. One of four black children in an all-white school, I was clearly unique. But since I'd always been told color was not a barrier, when I looked at everyone else, it wasn't the color of my skin that made me feel different. I walked into my classroom on the first day and what I saw was not a group of *white* children looking at me, but pairs and pairs of skinny legs all lined up at the back of the room. It's hard to believe, but I had no concept that I was different in any way except that I had *thighs* and they didn't. I burst into tears and ran out of the room.

For the next three days I sat in a corner of the principal's office, weeping silently to myself. On the fourth day, my sister convinced me to return to class, and she stayed with me until school was let out that afternoon. To my astonishment, the teacher and all my classmates were actually *nice* to me. Unlike these friendly first-graders, the community in which I lived was often hostile and violent. So, overwhelmed by this unexpected reception and somewhat recovered from the initial shock of all those skinny legs, on the fifth day I returned to the classroom all by myself.

More than anything I wanted to fit in at school, to be just like everyone else. My thick body prevented me from looking like the others, but I had no idea how to change my physical appearance. At suppertime I kept right on smothering my bread with butter, scooping gravy on my vegetables, and asking for a second helping of peach pie.

"How come your legs are so big?" a white girlfriend from class asked me one day. I told her I didn't know. "Well," she said, "when my momma gets too big, she goes on a lettuce diet. She won't eat anything but lettuce for days." This "dieting" was a new concept for me, but I was fascinated and said I'd try the lettuce diet, too. Suddenly it dawned on me: There was a direct connection between the food I ate and the size of my body! It wasn't long before I was hooked on dieting and losing weight; thus, the birth of a Diet Princess.

The lettuce diet paved the way for hundreds more to come. A large portion of my time and energy was spent worrying about getting fatter and dreaming up quick-weight-loss strategies. One strategy that proved effective was to be absent at mealtimes. Now that school provided the relief and comfort I needed in my life, mealtimes became less and less important. I'd dash off to school in the mornings before anyone noticed I hadn't eaten breakfast, and I'd purposely miss supper in the evenings, conjuring up dozens of excuses for having done so. When I heard about the "Grapefruit 45 Plan," I was so excited I consumed grapefruit after grapefruit at a frantic pace. One day I'd eaten so many grapefruits I had canker sores in my mouth and my stomach was so bloated I looked like a child from a poster depicting starvation victims. Once I read that eating an apple on an empty stomach could help me lose weight—the pectin was supposed to "significantly aid in the weight reduction process"—and so for days I ate nothing but apples. I lost weight, but my stamina also suffered. One afternoon, I was picking cherries from the top of a ladder and, suddenly, found myself flat on my back with my father staring down at me. I had blacked out at the top of the cherry tree, and it's a wonder I wasn't seriously hurt as I crashed down the rungs and onto the ground. Dazed, but also embarrassed when I realized what had happened, I told my father I had the flu and went home to bed.

By eleven, I had dieting down to a twisted science. I'd starve myself for days then, unable to control my hunger, I'd stuff anything I could find into my mouth. At one Fourth of July carnival, after two days of fasting, I suddenly turned into a living, breathing food vacuum. In less than two hours, I consumed three cotton candies, six corn dogs, two hamburgers, two orders of french fries, a sixteen-ounce bottle of Coke, one corn on the cob, four ice cream bars, and several bags of Peanut M&M's. Later, when I went home, I devoured half a chocolate cake and a quart of milk. Finally calling a halt to my feeding frenzy and in a near state of panic, I swallowed an entire box of laxatives and collapsed on my bed. My insides churned with pain, but this constant bingeing and purging had become my secret ritual. Always sick in bed the next day, I would hear my mother in the next room say, "Yep, Victoria must have the flu again. Wonder why she's so sick all the time . . ."

Adding to my self-image problems was the fact that physically, I matured much earlier than the other girls in my class. By the time I was in junior high school, my breasts were the size of melons and my thighs rubbed together when I walked down the hall. To compensate for my weight and also to satisfy an internal drive to succeed, I studied hard and joined in as many extracurricular activities as I could. I made the honor roll, I participated in theater, track, and dance. I was outgoing and popular, but my self-esteem and self-confidence remained low. When friends said to me, "You're such a fun person to be with," what I heard was, "You're such a fun *fat* person to be with."

About this time, my friends within the black community were suddenly beginning to distance themselves from me. By excelling at "white" subjects and showing enthusiasm for other school activities,

I was somehow demonstrating my rejection of black culture and black values, they felt. I was torn, on the one hand, by a fierce need to succeed and be the best, and on the other, by the strong cultural connections I had known all my life. I wasn't trying to be white or to reject my cultural heritage. I had simply found a community, namely my school and my new friends, which made me feel good and encouraged me to pursue my goals. Where did it say you could only be smart, fit and successful if you were white? I didn't believe it then and I don't believe it now. By fourteen my mind was made up: I would follow my dreams wherever they took me, no matter how far from home.

My family's financial situation slowly improved. When I was fifteen, we moved into our first real home a few blocks from the migrant workers' camp. Still obsessed with my weight, I worked as hard as I could to earn money for new weight loss devices and gimmicks, always hopeful that my next purchase would provide the "magic" cure. I did various jobs for neighbors and got involved in government-assisted programs that paid minimum wage to migrant students. I bought loofah sponges and rubbed my thighs until they were raw, but what I ended up with was nothing more than chafed fat. So, for months I saved my hard-earned dollars for a "Bubble Exercise Suit," a one-piece outfit I put on and connected to Mom's vacuum cleaner from a special opening in the back of the suit. The hot air circulating inside the bubble suit was supposed to help me sweat away my fat. What a ridiculous sight I must have been in that goofy bubble suit—the look of determination (mixed with terror) in my eyes, the sweat pouring down my cheeks, and the sound of the vacuum cleaner buzzing in my brain.

Despite my nonstop purchases, I knew that many of the newest and most "effective" fat-burning contraptions were accessible only in the expensive health clubs that I could never afford to join. Not about to let that stop me, I made my own modified versions of the gadgets at home. I had seen several pictures of rolling machines—big structures made with bars of grooved wood that you leaned up against to "roll" away your extra pounds. Thinking the rolling machines an impressive new invention, I devised my own using a wooden rolling pin from the kitchen. After my bath at night, I'd get out of the tub and frantically roll my stomach, hips, and thighs. When weeks of rolling my body produced no visible effects, I grudgingly returned the rolling pin to its rightful place in the cooking-utensil drawer.

The preoccupation with my weight continued, but one year a new passion developed after we were given a black-and-white television set by my father's boss: *dancing*. I loved watching *American Bandstand* and spent hours perfecting the dances I'd see on the shows. Now, in addition to saving for fat-removing devices, I started saving my money for dance shoes and dance lessons. I'd leave school early to sell apples during the day and then take classes at night to make up for missed time. My dancing ability enabled me to make the cheerleading squad that spring, but there were two strings attached: The cheerleading outfits cost $50, and the captain of the squad told me I needed to lose some weight before school started in the fall. To earn the $50 for my cheerleading outfit, I took on any odd job I could find, even working after dark stacking boxes in the rain. Desperate to lose the weight, I starved myself and abused laxatives and diet pills all summer long. I regularly took three times the recommended dosages, and as a result developed heart palpitations and became prone to frequent anxiety attacks. One hot August afternoon I collapsed and was rushed to the hospital for an emergency appendectomy. I returned home several days later severely depressed, with a huge scar across my stomach. My recovery was slow. I was still determined to be a cheerleader, but I had lost so much weight I was now too weak to make the practices. Eventually, I began eating again, and all the pounds (if not more) came back. By the end of the school year, my costly cheerleading outfit no longer fit.

Because of my overall enthusiasm for school and sports-related

activities, I also volunteered to be a P.E. assistant. When the instructor (whom I adored) became pregnant and could no longer teach
class, the job of teaching P.E. suddenly fell on my shoulders. No way
was I just going to make everyone do jumping jacks and sit-ups! I
began teaching the class dance routines and some of the movements
from cheerleading. When some of the teachers heard about my class,
they asked me to teach them in the evenings after school, too. They
all loved it, and so did I—but at that time I certainly wasn't thinking
of making a career of it!

After high school I attended various colleges in the area, and
wound up completing my studies in marketing and merchandising at
a private business college in Spokane, Washington. But I still yearned
to dance and was developing a real interest in exercise physiology
and nutrition, so I began taking night courses at a community college
nearby. I continued teaching aerobic dance classes (modified versions
of the P.E. classes) in the evenings to public-school teachers and
housewives, even though my weight climbed steadily toward 170
pounds. I talked to my students about good nutrition and health, but
I was a closet eater—a mass of contradictions (and a mass of fat).
Actually, my students told me they liked my class because I looked
just like them—I wasn't an intimidating instructor with a picture-
perfect body.

It had been almost fifteen years since the infamous lettuce diet,
and still I was convinced there was a miracle cure for my dieting
nightmare. No longer a Diet Princess, by this time I was a full-fledged
Diet Diva. I lived with one of my sisters in Spokane, and together we
concocted dozens of our own wild weight-loss schemes. If we hadn't
tried it, it was because it hadn't been invented yet. We went on the
protein diet, which requires that you eat nothing but protein for
weeks at a time. After four days of straight protein we were consti-
pated, light-headed, and slightly euphoric from ketosis, our "protein
high." We avoided body lotion and wore rubber gloves when we

cooked and did the dishes for fear the oils and fat could be absorbed into our bodies through our pores. I even tried "diet shots," which I later discovered were actually cow-placenta injections! Hopelessly bulimic, I continued consuming huge quantities of food, only to force all of it from my body by immediately making myself throw up or swallowing my stand-by package of laxatives.

In 1981, an aerobics craze was sweeping the country, and in no time it had swept me up, too: I decided to make fitness and health my full-time career. Though I was noticeably overweight, my aerobics classes were popular. I was praised for my energy, devotion, and enthusiasm. Then one day I overheard one of my students say, "Victoria moves pretty good for a fat chick." The comment devastated me. Desperately wanting to lose my extra pounds, I sought counseling to help me understand and control my eating disorder, I attended nationally based weight loss programs, and called Overeaters Anonymous Hot Lines constantly (good thing they were toll-free numbers, or I'd have gone broke!). But still the behavior continued. At home I devoured entire pepperoni pizzas, bags of Doritos, and batches of chocolate-chip cookies, only to whine about it during counseling sessions later. As if possessed, I drove from McDonald's to Burger King to Wendy's inhaling Big Macs, french fries, and chocolate shakes, trying to time my stops so the same employee wouldn't recognize me at the drive-up window an hour later.

After years of insane dieting, of bingeing and purging, I was beginning to think my covert eating rituals would always be a part of my life. Then I began regularly experiencing fainting spells and dizziness. I was tired all the time and yet I couldn't sleep at night. A friend convinced me to make an emergency appointment with her doctor. Physically I knew I was a mess, but it wasn't until the doctor's appointment that I discovered the real damage I'd inflicted upon my body over the years. It proved to be a major turning point in my life, and I can remember certain events from the visit as clearly as if it had happened yesterday . . .

The first thing the nurse did was ask me to step on the scale. I knew I'd probably put on a few pounds, but I usually avoided scales and so didn't really know how much I weighed at that point. I dropped my purse, took off my shoes, my earrings—anything to make me weigh less. She began adjusting the scale. First she set it at 120 pounds, then 130 pounds, then 140, then 150, then 160, then 170 . . . She was about to go further, but at 170 pounds I jumped off the scale and began screaming, "Oh, my God! Oh, my God!" My arm whacked the nurse's folder and her papers flew all over the office. A second nurse rushed over to help calm me down. I was sobbing; I had totally lost control. It was as if the world was coming to an end.

Besides my being grossly overweight, the checkup also revealed the following: My pancreas was barely functional, I had a heart murmur, and my electrolytes were out of balance. The doctor also told me I needed to get a handle on my diet because I was borderline diabetic. (As if those things weren't enough, a few weeks later a dentist discovered that my jaw was deteriorating and some of my teeth had begun to crumble. At some point I would require extensive oral surgery.)

One thought finally hit home that day: If I didn't make the commitment to change my behavior once and for all, it was clear I would eventually destroy myself.

Attitude Adjustment

After seeing the dial on the scale hit 170 pounds and after being told I'd probably develop diabetes in the near future, I realized I couldn't run from the truth any longer. That afternoon the doctor and I had a long discussion about my past and about my bulimia. In the end, he told me what I already knew but had always avoided thinking about:

that my problems with food stemmed from the many violent and tragic memories I had been carrying around since childhood; early on, eating had become my primary means of comfort, and as I grew I carried that food/comfort association with me right into adulthood. My problems were not only physical at this point, they were definitely psychological as well. Now it was time to let go and allow the healing process to begin.

Trapped for years in a deadly binge/purge cycle, thinking myself incurable and alone in my suffering from such a bizarre relationship with food, I decided, finally, *enough is enough*. That afternoon I deliberately drove a new route home, bypassing the familiar fast-food restaurants with their glaring golden arches and brightly painted burgers, those old "friends" who could so easily lure me to the drive-up window . . . "Hey, Victoria, how about a cheeseburger or two? Large fries? A chocolate shake?" It was time to break the destructive habits that in part perpetuated such a vicious cycle of overeating. By avoiding my fast-food haunts that day, I had taken a small, positive step toward change.

Over the next few days, I thought again about some of the life-enhancing techniques and strategies that I had learned from various courses over the years. I started setting some goals for myself. First, I *had* to do something about the deteriorating condition of my health, which I knew meant changing what and how I ate. Second, I decided to set a professional goal: to become an influential force within the fitness community and to spread my passion for aerobics and physical fitness throughout the country. Last, I wanted to learn how to look at my reflection in the mirror and like the person I saw—the most important, but also the most difficult goal to achieve. These were my long-term goals; I had no delusions about accomplishing them overnight. I had finally realized there was no such thing as a "quick fix."

Beyond just establishing my goals, the next step was to take some positive action. (I had also taken enough goal-setting classes in the past to know that without the follow-up action, goal setting was useless.) I moved to Portland, Oregon, shortly thereafter to pursue business opportunities in fitness and to gain further experience in the field of aerobics. During my last four years of teaching students and instructors in Spokane, it became obvious that I needed to move to a larger metropolitan area where the market for aerobics was greater. Plus, my workshops were much more in demand farther south in Seattle and Los Angeles. Portland seemed like a nice compromise, but eventually I hoped to make it all the way down to Los Angeles.

I began absorbing all the information I could about fitness and health. I enrolled in various programs that took me from Wichita, where I studied exercise science, nutritional biochemistry, and athletic training, to Dallas, where I became a certified instructor through the American Council on Exercise (ACE) and the Aerobic Fitness Association of America (AFAA), both of which represent continuing education in the field of aerobic fitness (and whose courses I now teach). I studied under Covert Bailey, the author of *Fit or Fat*, and became licensed to teach his program. After completing these courses, I began working with the Northwest Aerobic Association and continued to increase my knowledge about exercise science, kinesiology, sports medicine, and the biomechanics of proper exercise. In the midst of my educational splurge, I became inspired by Dr. Kenneth Cooper's book, *The Aerobics Program for Total Well-being*, and took up power walking and distance running. Dr. Cooper, the recognized "father of aerobics," touted the benefits of running long distances at a slower pace (versus running shorter distances at faster speeds). To me, a former high-school sprinter, this was an entirely new approach to running. He determined that running long slow distances would increase one's endurance level plus burn a higher percentage of fat. *Burn more fat?* I was sold: Time to hit the pavement! I began running or walking every other day, and in a few months' time my endurance level improved, some of my extra pounds vanished, and my aerobics classes became more effective. In addition to teaching at a health club, I formed my own company to educate and train aerobics instructors while at the same time promoting a weight-control program that offered body-fat testing, nutritional advice, and personal training. Dr. Cooper was so much of an inspiration that I also got certified through his Institute of Aerobic Research.

Although I was making significant progress toward my professional goal, changing my eating habits proved much more of a challenge. In order to change the way I ate, I needed to change my mind-set about food—I needed to change the way I *thought* about food. But how? Having studied nutrition previously, I knew basically what kinds of foods my body did and did not need. Anxious to learn more, I frequented the popular diet centers and attended local hospital programs on dieting, weight management, and nutrition. Clearly my problem wasn't that I lacked information; my problem was that I lacked motivation and control over my eating. I lacked *personal power*. While I knew I had to change, mentally I just wasn't committed to getting the results I desired. And I had all the excuses down, too: from "I'm too busy to fix dinner tonight," to "I'm too tired to go grocery shopping," to "Oh, one more order of french fries isn't going to hurt me." Once again I saw counselors who specialized in eating disorders, and as a result did experience occasional success in sticking with a healthy nutritional regimen. But most days I abandoned technical knowledge (not to mention common sense) altogether, and the binges and purges continued.

At this point my weight simply plateaued at 150 pounds; I had stopped gaining weight, but I had also stopped losing it—no matter what I did. Then one day I noticed someone new at the health club where I worked: a personal trainer and champion bodybuilder named Davis McGinty. A massive 245 pounds of pure muscle, Davis was instructing a small group of women in some of the methods and techniques used by professional bodybuilders. Part teddy bear, part drill sergeant, Davis pushed these women to work out as hard as they could and yet also managed effectively to motivate and encourage them. They took their workouts seriously, but they obviously enjoyed them, too. Most importantly, they were getting *results*. I began regularly observing their sessions together, and in a few weeks *all* the women had begun to change the shape of their bodies. Single-handedly, this man was turning marshmallows into rocks, soft bodies into hard bodies. Here I was on my exercise bike, pedaling my buns off for an hour every day, not to mention leaping around the aerobics room like a crazy woman, and still *my* body looked like a large pear. What were they doing that I wasn't? What did they know that I didn't? Anxious to find out, I set up an appointment with Davis the following day.

To my complete surprise, Davis told me a few things I'll never forget: "Victoria, with all the aerobic training you're doing right now you probably have the world's strongest heart. But, honey, if you want to change those thighs and those arms, you're gonna have to pump some iron!" He told me I had potential as a bodybuilder because of my strong legs (they *should* have been strong, carrying around forty extra pounds for all those years!), and that with his help I could lose weight and permanently change the shape of my body. My first thought was, "Yeah, sure. You're talkin' to the *Diet Diva* here, mister. What makes you think you've got all the answers?" On the other hand, I was impressed by his success with the other women; their leaner, stronger bodies were positive proof he knew what he was doing. I handed him a check, and we went to work.

During our first few sessions Davis taught me basic bodybuilding techniques and put me on a six-meal eating plan, a strict diet of low-fat foods consisting of moderate amounts of complex carbohydrates and protein, and minute traces of fat. He made me keep a detailed journal in which I wrote about everything from what I ate to what I felt throughout the day to what my sleep patterns were at night.

Davis set the basic format for the journal, and I personalized it with information about myself. Knowing I would be accountable to this man every week was probably the most motivating factor in this whole process. But, I still gave *him* the ultimate responsibility for changing my body because psychologically I didn't feel strong enough to do it alone. The journal I kept was important because it helped me keep a clear, constant picture of my thoughts and behavior—those things that were keeping me from reaching my goals and keeping me from adopting new, healthier, more empowering thoughts and behavior patterns.

If I ever expected to change my physical appearance, first I would have to change some basic beliefs about myself. In the past, I really did not believe I could ever lose weight. Then again, maybe I really didn't *want* to lose the weight. Maybe my weight was a defense mechanism designed to keep men away from me. My experiences had taught me that women were powerless when it came to men, so maybe I was afraid of becoming too attractive. If men never came (or wanted to come) near me, then I couldn't get hurt by them. Whatever my reasons, it was very difficult for me to visualize a lean, thin Victoria. Through my work with Davis, I eventually began to see myself in a new light, and I began behaving in ways that brought me closer to my new image of a strong, lean Victoria, a woman in control of her life. In the end, how I envisioned myself and what I believed about myself was eventually how I came to be.

In no time I was totally consumed with bodybuilding. I was *pumped up!* I attended special weight-training camps and nutritional seminars, all the while setting my sights on actually competing someday. I pictured myself on stage in a skimpy bikini, flexing my oiled muscles and grinning at the crowd. A bodybuilder friend once told me, "If it moves, it's yours, so make sure the right things are moving up there." By the end of one year, I was a new person. The "right things" were definitely moving. My weight had dropped from 150 to

114 pounds, and my body fat went from 28 percent to 10 percent. The health problems that my doctor had discovered several years earlier had all but vanished.

To this day I still train off and on with Davis, and I believe he played a major role in helping me change my physical appearance as well as teaching me about personal strength and power. To progress to the point where I could bench-press 145 pounds (not bad for a woman once shaped like a pear!) made me feel strong and confident. Davis used to say to me, "Who do you want this bar to be? Push it out of your way! *Move it!* When you set that bar back down, leave that person out there away from your body, out of your mind's eye, away from your emotional sights. With each lift, that person moves farther and farther away. Pretty soon he or she will be completely gone."

Realistically I knew I couldn't expect my personal trainer to keep tabs on my food intake and my muscle tone forever; at some point I knew the responsibility would ultimately be mine. After I stopped training regularly with Davis, I began looking for ways to help myself maintain my new physique and life-style. I had experienced many successes in the past two years, but I hadn't really learned to like myself, and I worried constantly about losing my motivation and slipping back into my bad habits of the past, not to mention putting the weight back on again. Although it was true I had a new body, I didn't quite have a new *attitude* yet.

I searched my own subconscious mind for some positive internal tapes, and I remembered some of the marketing meetings and rallies I'd gone to several years back. Back then I had had no desire to sell soap or vitamin products, but I *was* impressed by the hype and hoopla of those sessions. Recalling all the "Rah, rah, rah, you can do it" and "Go get 'em" talk, I wondered how I could begin permanently applying that kind of enthusiasm to my own life. Once again I attended motivational seminars and workshops (I spent over $4,800 that year!); I read all the latest books on motivation, self-esteem, and self-concept. I even listened to self-improvement cassettes while I drove. I practiced visualization techniques, described my feelings and worked out my problems on the pages of countless journals. In retrospect, I was fine-tuning my attitude.

Finally, I was ready to tell others what I had learned. Though I had changed *my life* over the past two years, I knew there were many other people who needed to be taught how to erase their pains and how to feel good about themselves, how to lead happier, more fulfilled lives. I felt that this, combined with teaching about good health and physical fitness, was my *mission*. Exercise had always been a positive force in my life. Through all the physical movement, the sweat and laughter that accompanied my own workouts as well as my teaching, I gained confidence, renewed enthusiasm, and ultimately inner strength and peace. I thought that if exercise could make me feel this good, why couldn't it do the same for others?

Exercise *can* make you feel this good, and you don't have to take hundreds of classes, hire a personal trainer, or become a professional aerobics instructor to learn how, either. That was what I felt I needed to teach others, and it's what I'll be showing *you* how to accomplish in this book.

"And the rest," as they say, "is history." Well, almost. Sure, I've come a long way since my bubble suit days. But the truth is, I'm really just like you. I'm still working, still struggling, still battling my insecurities, still resisting urges to binge, and still doing my best to drown out those old negative tapes playing in my head. I haven't "made it"; I haven't "arrived" anywhere. My journey continues. Learning and recovering is a lifelong process—we're always in training.

Chapter Two:
Life Training

Your Turn

All of us have our own stories to tell—our own family backgrounds and histories, our own triumphs and failures, our own joys and passions, our own pains and disappointments, our own problems to solve. Sometimes these problems are in the forefront of our minds; sometimes they become nagging concerns that occasionally creep up to the surface and manage to upset us or make us feel guilty. Some problems are real, some are imagined but all of them affect the way we feel and behave. Because of certain events in our lives, some of us have pains that go much, much deeper. Unwilling to acknowledge these wounds, let alone try to repair them, we become workaholics, exercise fanatics, anorexics, and bulimics. We seek relief through such destructive forms of behavior as drinking and drug abuse, or any number of escape routes available to us. Though they may provide temporary comfort and relief, in the long run these avoidance tactics only magnify our problems and take us even further away from a healthy recovery.

For years I was in a similar state of denial. I was looking for external miracles instead of internal strength, which is what led to my bingeing and purging. During my senior year in high school I was voted "Best Personality," but no one really knew the pain I felt or the hurt I was hiding inside. My classmates came from comfortable homes and wore beautiful new clothes to school; I lived in a virtual shack, shared a bedroom with five of my brothers and sisters, and wore clothes that had been passed down several times after having been purchased secondhand to begin with. How could they know my pain when I hid it so well from myself?

Although our pasts are important in terms of who and where we are today, the fact is that we cannot change what happened to us five, ten, twenty years ago. Fortunately, we *can* change where we're going tomorrow, and that's what this chapter is about: creating a lifelong game plan for healthy, effective living. This chapter is a course in *life training*.

I'll bet this is not the first time you've purchased a health, fitness, or diet-related book. Am I right? If so, what did you do with the last one you bought? Did you read it cover to cover? Did you really make an effort to incorporate its principles and techniques into your life-style? Did you become more physically fit, lose weight, improve your internal tapes, reach your goals? I recently learned from a book publisher that fewer than 10 percent of the health and fitness books purchased are ever read all the way through. Not surprising, given the fact that fewer than 5 percent of all the people in America who lose weight actually manage to *keep* the weight off (as a former Diet Diva, I can certainly relate to that statistic!).

If you're like most people, you want quick, easy results. You want instant gratification. I wanted to take a pill that would make my fat disappear overnight. Guess what? It never happened. I didn't find the solution overnight; I found it *over time*. Real change and healing doesn't happen overnight; in most cases the change and recovery process is never ending. You fall off the wagon from time to time, you occasionally lose sight of your goals. Okay, so you're human. *The key*

▼

You can't change yester-

day, but you can control

tomorrow.

is not to abandon your journey. Don't beat yourself up mentally, just get back on the life training program. It's taken me years to reach the point where I am today, to feel in control of my life and to live *my attitude*. Still, I know I'll never be completely "cured"; I'll never be completely healed. As long as negative forces exist (and they will), I'll always be fighting the urge to overeat. But perfection isn't a realistic goal for anyone. What's important is that as you go through life, you begin learning from your experiences and begin thinking of them as opportunities for growth, not self-defeat. When new opportunities arise, you respond to them, you meet them head-on. The quicker you deal with them, the quicker you'll find a solution.

You know my story; now it's *your* turn.

Give Yourself a Big Hand!

In the previous chapter, I told you about my past and how one particularly revealing visit to the doctor's office finally made me commit to changing my unhealthy, destructive behavior patterns. It's time now to focus on yourself—on the positive aspects of your life as well as those aspects you'd like to change. By demonstrating the simple techniques I used back then, you will learn how to begin making the changes you desire in your own life. Think of the rest of these pages as a workbook dedicated to your personal growth and development. Make a commitment to yourself. You're worth it!

Psychologists have known for years that in order to change negative thoughts and behavior you must engage in positive "self talk" (remember those internal tapes I spoke of at the beginning of the book?). When you were a child, chances are your parents encouraged you to revel in and feel proud of your accomplishments. As an adult, however, you've been taught to cheer for others but never for yourself. The older you've become, the less "cool" it is to clap for yourself. Well,

I think it's time to reinstate the concept of *self-praise*. Don't confuse my meaning here: I'm not talking about developing an inflated ego; I'm not encouraging you to walk around projecting things like "Don't you wish *you* looked like me?" or "My kids are better than your kids!" There's a big difference between insecure ego projection and positive self-talk: one makes other people feel inferior, the other affirms your sense of self-worth without hurting anyone else in the process.

Part of why I struggled with eating disorders and low self-esteem for so many years was because I never took the time to acknowledge those things about myself that *were* positive, those things I did that made me feel good. All I could see were the numbers on the scale. I went overboard in terms of applauding others, but I never took the time to pat myself on the back or praise myself for anything. Now I know you *must* learn to cheer for yourself—I mean, if *you* don't, who will? Learn to become your own best cheerleader.

These days I always tell my students at the end of a class, "Give yourselves a big hand! You did fantastic today!" When I first started saying this to them, most students stared at me as if I'd lost my mind.

The next time I said it they clapped quietly, then exited the room as quickly as possible. Now they cheer and clap loudly for themselves because it makes them feel good and they're no longer embarrassed by those words. They're proud of themselves, and they should be. My students are some of the greatest people in the world!

In the spaces below, give *yourself* a big hand.

FOUR OF MY BEST QUALITIES ARE:

(Examples: I am a hard worker; I have a great smile; I have beautiful handwriting; I'm honest.)
(It doesn't matter how big or how small you feel your strong points are, just know that they're all significant.)

1.

2.

3.

4.

▼

One ounce of criticism needs one pound of compliments to balance the scale. Think good thoughts about yourself.

Yes! You should feel good about those attributes! It's important to remember these positive qualities, especially when the negative tapes start running through your head.

Negative Forces Require Positive Responses

Okay. It's time to face the bad guys. Take a moment to think about your problems—the areas of your life that need improving, the negative kinds of behavior you want to change, what's hurting you that you want to get rid of. This isn't easy; I know that. Facing reality and admitting you have problems takes courage. Recognition and admission are the hardest part of the healing process, but they're also the crucial first step. . . .

FOUR THINGS I NEED TO
CHANGE/IMPROVE ABOUT MYSELF ARE:

(Examples: I want to learn to accept myself; I want to learn better ways of controlling my anger; I want to become more physically fit.)

1.

2.

3.

4.

The next step is to determine what negative thoughts or emotions are keeping you from making the changes you want. Ask yourself, "What is it that's preventing me from making the changes I desire? What self-defeating thoughts do I need to eliminate? What internal tapes do I need to eject?" When you've identified the most common ones, write them below.

FOUR THOUGHTS OR EMOTIONS THAT PREVENT ME FROM CHANGING ARE:

(Examples: I'm afraid I'll fail; I'll never be good enough; I'm afraid what others will think; I'm not ready yet.)

1.

2.

3.

4.

These thoughts and emotions can be paralyzing. They can mentally cripple you or stop you dead in your tracks. Be aware of their existence and question their validity. Make every conscious effort to replace these negative tapes with positive new ones.

Just because you've always thought something about yourself is true doesn't mean it is true.

As with any negative force in your life, be it a destructive form of behavior, a nagging, self-defeating thought, or a problematic person, you must develop ways of *responding* positively, not *reacting* negatively. *Responding* to a thought, a situation, or a person entails gaining control of your feelings by stepping back emotionally and/or physically, closing your eyes, breathing rhythmically, and questioning and assessing the experience in a calm, rational way. Don't set yourself up for more trouble by immediately *reacting* to the negative forces. That bottle of vodka isn't going to help, and neither is that carton of ice cream. Remember, it's not what happens to you in life, it's how you *think* about what happens that really matters. Likewise, how you *choose* to respond to the negative forces will determine whether or not you'll come out a winner. The winner, by the way, is the one who stays focused on the desired outcome and remains in control.

Rethink the last situation you were involved in that made you feel powerless, hurt, frustrated, disappointed, scared, nervous, angry, jealous, sad. Was it something someone said or was it the way someone looked at you? Who made you feel this way: your mother, father, spouse, child, boss, friend, a complete stranger? Now try to remember how you reacted to your emotions. Did you react by hurting the person in return, eating a box of chocolates, or crying yourself to sleep that night? How could you respond more effectively next time? Sometimes you need to listen quietly, sometimes you simply need to leave the room until your anger has subsided. You're unique and you need to discover what works best for you, but it helps to think about your initial reactions so you won't repeat them the next time.

When I was ten years old, I performed a lip-sync dance routine in a talent contest and *won*. Afterward, I felt so good about myself, so proud and confident. I just knew I was destined for Broadway—no one could have convinced me otherwise. To this day, whenever I feel insecure or feel my confidence slipping away, I go back in my memory to an internal tape labeled "Talent Show." I imagine that the people judging me presently are the same ones who judged my routine at the talent show. Before I know it, I experience those same feelings of strength and self-assurance; I'm able to shut out my fears and insecurities and focus on getting the job done. Develop a positive-recall system like this and try it out the next time you're overwhelmed by negative, self-critical thoughts.

Think positively and be strong. Make a plan, rehearse your responses, know what you want the outcome to be.

No one likes to admit to having problems or to being out of control. But you know what? The only people without problems are *dead* people. (Not a pleasant alternative, if you ask me.) Happy, successful people don't have fewer problems than you; they simply respond more positively and therefore solve their problems more effectively. To begin with, why not try changing how you *think* about your problems? Instead of viewing them as defeats, try looking at them as challenges and as opportunities for personal growth. You'll be amazed what a simple change in *attitude* can do.

▼

The only power that people and situations have over you is the power that you give them.

10 KEYS TO PROBLEM SOLVING

1. Consciously recognize the problem; meet it head-on, then deal with it. If you can't solve it right away, come back to it later.

2. Write it down, commit it to paper. Sometimes seeing it on paper reduces its size and impact. Break it down; see it for what it really is.

3. Don't blame others. Take personal responsibility for your life.

4. View the problem objectively; yours isn't the only point of view. Don't be afraid to say "I screwed up," if in fact you did.

5. Get creative—explore every possible solution. Ignore obstacles in your path; look for hurdles you can jump over, not walls you have to tear down.

6. Organize the solutions. Enthusiasm is great, but don't create another problem through overzealous reactions. Make a plan and take it one step at a time.

7. Ask for advice from someone you trust. You don't have to have all the answers; no one does. The president has a cabinet. Most companies have boards of directors. Don't let your personal pride stand in the way of your successful future.

8. Learn from previous problems and behavior. Don't repeat the past. Anticipate potential problems and plan your responses ahead of time.

9. Stay in control and keep a winning attitude.

10. Most important, be true to yourself. Know your outcome.

No More Excuses!

As I tell my students, "It's time to jam, y'all!" I'm telling you the same thing, so let's get busy! You've already identified your problems and the behavior patterns you'd like to change, and you've learned some techniques for dealing with all the negative forces in your life. Next, you need to set your goals and establish a game plan for yourself. Goals are a vital part of everyday life: They inspire and motivate you to be your best; they are what will determine your success or your failure in life. You need both short-term and long-term goals, and they should be written down, tracked, evaluated, reassessed, and rewritten on a regular basis.

First, your goals must be action oriented and specific, and should include target dates. It's important that you have a clear picture in your mind of what it is you want to accomplish. For example, if your general goal is to *exercise*, you probably won't do it. Your goal needs to be more specific, more focused. Here's an example of a more focused goal: "I want to exercise regularly so I'll live longer, have more energy, and have a healthy retirement." Another might be: "I want to exercise to lose weight and to change the shape of my body." See what I mean? The more specific you can be with your goals, the more incentive you'll have and the greater your chances of actually reaching your goals.

Second, set goals that are realistic, attainable, and measurable. If your goal is to improve your level of cardiovascular fitness and to change the shape of your body but you want to do it in three months' time, ask yourself if this is reasonable. Do you really have the motivation and can you devote the hours that it will take to accomplish your goal? If not, try starting on a smaller scale. Build up to your goals, but remember to acknowledge and reward yourself for those smaller successes along the way, too—they're important.

MY SHORT-TERM GOALS ARE:

(Examples: I will lose 10 pounds in 4 months; At the end of 6 weeks I'll be more organized; In 2 months I will gain 2 pounds of muscle.)

1.

2.

3.

MY LONG-TERM GOALS ARE:

(Examples: I will lose 20 pounds in 1 year; In 6 months all the closets in my house will be organized; By this time next year I will be exercising 4 times a week.)

1.

2.

3.

Is what you're doing today bringing you any closer to where you want to be tomorrow? Think about it.

You've identified *what* your goals are, now let's work on *how* you're going to make them happen. To accomplish your goals, you need to develop a game plan; you must establish specific *actions* to take. If your goal over the next twelve months is to improve your cardiovascular fitness and change the shape of your body, your plan of action might include taking an hour-long aerobics class three times a week and training with weights for two days. On the other hand, such a routine might be too much to ask of yourself initially. Instead, try walking during your noon hour and attending an aerobics class on the weekend. Purchase a pair of hand weights or exercise bands and go through some of the routines in the section on body sculpting (page 201) while you're watching TV at night. Remember: What works for someone else may not work for you, so don't start comparing yourself with anyone else. You are unique and special. Personalize your plan. Make it work for *you*.

Some of the goals you've set up for yourself may be based on changing unhealthy behavior patterns or self-defeating thoughts that have been going on for a long time. If so, you may need to reach out into your community for help. Consult your physician or employee-assistance programs at work. Check the phone book for groups or organizations that might be able to assist you, or at least point you in the right direction. Your plan of action may be as simple at first as looking in the yellow pages for support-group therapy. After receiving the necessary information, however, study it and then set new goals for yourself, like planning to attend specific programs or classes available in your area.

As I mentioned before, change is a progressive, lifelong training process—don't expect miracles overnight. Start today by setting realistic goals for yourself and then following through with concrete action. Stay focused. Before long, you will have internalized the process; it will become habit, a positive part of you.

HERE'S YOUR GAME PLAN:

▲ SHORT-TERM GOAL
(Example: Lose 5 pounds in 2 months.)

1.

2.

3.

▲ ACTION
(Example: Cut fat intake and walk daily.)

1.

2.

3.

▲ LONG-TERM GOAL
(Example: Get my business life organized.)

1.

2.

3.

▲ ACTION
(Examples: Buy a daily planner; discuss subject with colleagues.)

1.

2.

3.

▼

All thoughts create actions; all actions create habits; all habits create results.

See It

An important part of the goal-setting process is the practice of daily visualization. Visualization is the act of picturing your goal in your mind's eye and then seeing yourself actually accomplishing that goal. Let's say you want to learn to control your anger. Close your eyes and imagine yourself in a situation that might normally cause you to blow up. Instead of slamming your fist down on the table or hurling a book across the room, see yourself taking a deep breath, then removing yourself from the situation and returning to it only when you're capable of responding in a more constructive manner. If you want to lose twenty-five pounds, picture yourself shopping and browsing through a rack of dresses two sizes smaller than what you wear now. See yourself marching off to the dressing room with an armload of dresses, then standing in front of the mirror watching yourself zip up each one. They fit perfectly—yes! You're rehearsing the result, trying it on in your mind.

Try using visualization techniques every day. I do, and I'm not alone. Athletes visualize everything from making the winning basket, to sinking the impossible putt, to landing the triple axel. Some actually *see* the outcome on the scoreboard or *feel* the gold medal hanging around their neck. The more clearly you can picture yourself reaching your goal, the more your subconscious mind believes that what you're seeing is the real thing. At some point it's so convinced that what you see is true, suddenly you're not just *imagining* you're a size six anymore; the size-six dress is on your body and you're walking down the street! Your vision has become a reality. See it, believe it, and eventually you'll live it.

▼

The more vividly you see yourself reaching your goals, the greater your chances of actually realizing them.

Write It Down

For many years, food constituted my escape route. When the going got tough, when I became depressed or angry, I'd immediately raid the cupboards, the refrigerator, or the freezer, inhaling anything and everything. Afterward, I'd panic and frantically try to rid my body of the thousands of calories I'd just consumed. Not only was I unwilling to commit to changing my destructive behavior, but I was also unable to deal with my problems in a constructive manner.

Today, one of the ways I deal with my problems and my feelings is to write about them. I keep countless journals, but if they're not handy I'll grab any piece of paper and write nonstop about what's bothering me. In the process of writing everything down, somehow I begin to see things more clearly, I become more relaxed and able to address the problem effectively. I may save what I've written, or I may wad it up in a ball and throw it in the trash; for me, that's like throwing away the problem. Either way, writing my thoughts down on paper makes a lot more sense than devouring an entire bag of potato chips or a package of cookies.

Though you may not be used to it, start keeping a journal. Use it to keep track of how you're progressing with your goals or to record certain thoughts and feelings. Use your journal to prevent you from reacting in negative ways and calling up negative emotions. Don't reach for a candy bar, reach for a piece of paper. Remember your positive qualities and recall happy memories, remember your successes and reaffirm your goals. After a few months' time, go back and read what you've written. What's changed since those first entries? What have you learned about yourself since then? Look how far you've come! This is part of your life training. It never ends. Remember: He who stays in the race, finishes.

▼

Are you in life training,

or death preparation?

Make It Happen!

I told you it was my personal goal with this book to inspire you and to help you change the quality of your life, and in this chapter I've shown you how you can go about making those changes you desire. Still, *all of this information is useless if you don't apply it or commit to taking action.* Don't be another losing statistic; be a winner, take control! It's up to you to make your life a success. Don't repeat the cycle of "Motivated and strong today, unmotivated and weak tomorrow." Take your first step today and remain focused tomorrow. Remember how the railroad system was built? One tie at a time. Keep building your own road to successful living one tie at a time, and don't take your foot off that track!

▼

Life is not a rehearsal— give your best performance every day!

LIFE TRAINING TIPS

1. Become your own best cheerleader; if you don't believe in yourself, who will?
2. Eliminate the negative self-talk from your vocabulary and your subconscious mind.
3. Respond positively to negative forces; begin viewing your life's problems as opportunities for personal growth and development, not as opportunities to fail.
4. Develop a game plan for yourself: Set goals and determine which actions will bring you closer to your desired results.
5. Who you see is who you'll be: Practice visualization techniques.
6. Put it on paper. Keep a regular journal.
7. You can choose to lose, or you can choose to win: The choice is yours.
8. Stay on track. Never give up!

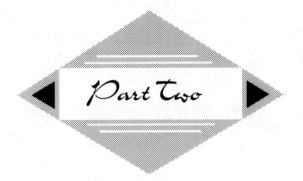

Part Two

LIVE

TO EAT, OR EAT

TO LIVE?

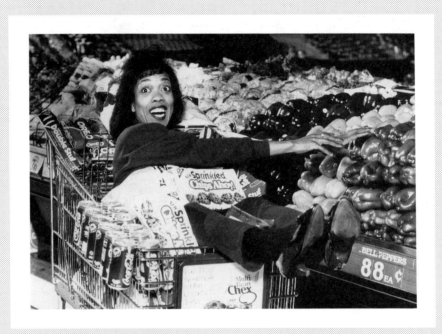

Chapter Three:
How Well Does Your Engine Run?

Up to this point I've given you many tools and techniques for evaluating your present state of thinking and behaving, and I've given you formulas for creating a more positive focus and direction for your life. Although all these things are intended to be inspiring and challenging, none of them matters unless you have the energy to get up off your behind, grab a pen, and actually begin formulating your self-improvement game plan. How is your energy level these days? Are you constantly fatigued and unmotivated? Do you wake up exhausted even after eight hours of sleep? Are you one of those people who carries around a lot of good intentions and new resolutions but never quite gets to the follow-through stage? Why is that? Hmm . . . Remember that old saying, "The spirit is willing but the flesh is weak?" Is this where you're at right now—too tired to get up off the couch and move across the room? Too weak to take action?

When people come to me complaining of constant fatigue, irritability, headaches, a lack of energy, and no motivation, the first thing I ask them is, "What kinds of food are you eating?" All moving things require energy or fuel, and your body gets its energy from the food you eat. Food is the fuel that makes your engine run, and the quality of that fuel determines the quality of your engine's performance. If you eat healthy, nutritious foods, your body will obtain all the energy it needs for optimum performance of all your daily tasks—both physical and mental. On the other hand, if you don't eat well, you won't perform well. In some cases you won't even perform at all: After a meal you'll just plop yourself down on the couch, turn on the TV, or take a nap, thus allowing all the garbage you just ate to really go to work on your system, leaving its debris in your arteries and around your waistline.

Eating right is serious business. What you eat determines how successfully you'll function today, and it determines how healthy you'll be tomorrow. You can choose to eat foods that benefit your body, or you can choose to keep eating junk. But in my mind, your choice of foods is just as important as whom you choose for president: After all, *both* affect your future!

My past food choices were horrible. My engine never had a chance to perform properly because it was always clogged up with sugar, salt, and fat. You don't believe me? Take a look. . . .

▼

"Life itself is the proper binge." (Julia Child)

A System Overhaul

I grew up in a community that, for the most part, encouraged heavy eating and didn't wince at the sight of a large body. Being overweight wasn't viewed negatively; it meant you weren't poor, you weren't starving, and your basic needs were being met. But the fact is, we were poor. Not only that, the starchy, high-fat farm diet we consumed was terrible for us. It wasn't until I became self-conscious about my weight in my early elementary-school years that I began to question some of these basic premises surrounding food and make some of my own decisions about my diet and appearance. Up to that point, I was basically eating on autopilot—eating without thinking, one binge after another.

All my bad eating habits began when I was a young child. At 4:00

A.M. the family was up and ready to go to work in the fields. Before heading out, I'd usually eat some of the following: a handful of crackers, a peanut-butter sandwich, cheese I carved off a huge block we received from government programs, or a fried-egg sandwich made from a powdered-egg mix I glopped between two pieces of white bread. When we returned from the fields around 7:30 A.M., my mother prepared a large breakfast of fried eggs, bacon (or some kind of canned meat we got from the welfare office), biscuits made with lard, and oatmeal covered with butter, sugar, and condensed milk. By the time I left for school, I had already consumed enough fat and calories for the rest of the day!

For lunch I ate whatever was served in the school cafeteria: greasy main courses of toasted cheese sandwiches, chili, lasagna, tacos, fried chicken, and mashed potatoes topped with gravy. My favorite, however, were "pigs in a blanket"—hot dogs wrapped in crescent rolls and melted cheese. "Fat wrapped in crap" would have been a more accurate description, I'm sure. Canned vegetables and fruit always came with these "entrees," and for dessert I ate doughnuts, cinnamon rolls, cakes, pies, or cookies. So much for watching my salt and sugar intake!

After school, if I wasn't involved in any extracurricular activities like cheerleading or track, I was back in the fields harvesting. While I picked fruit, I munched on nuts or candy I'd stuffed in my pockets. Sometimes I carried bags of chips or cookies along with me which I'd leave next to a tree or at the end of a row, using them as my reward for having filled a lot of baskets or completed a certain row. Though the work was tiring, I always looked forward to this time of day because it meant spending time with my family laughing, joking, and listening to more of my father's stories.

But the real "nightmare on 'E' Street" (my old street address) occurred after I came home from the fields at night, which was 7:30 P.M. An hour later, after I'd cleaned up and my mother had fixed supper, I feasted on fried chicken, red beans and rice, cornbread (like the biscuits, prepared with lard), yams served with butter, Kool-Aid with extra tablespoons of sugar, whole milk, and chocolate cake and ice cream for dessert. After polishing off two large helpings, I'd continue to snack on leftovers or some other kind of sweets as I finished my homework and got ready for bed.

Except for the times when I was dieting or fasting, these eating patterns remained basically the same until I left home after high school. But even when I was dieting I still fell into strict routines that never varied despite the physical problems that often developed as a result. (Remember the all-grapefruit diet that gave me canker sores and a cramped, bloated stomach?)

When I left home for college, suddenly I was on my own and free to choose my own meals. My former eating habits changed, but they were replaced by ones equally as bad. After I started teaching aerobics in the mornings, I stopped eating breakfast altogether (a big mistake!). By the time my class was over, I was famished and dashed to McDonald's hoping to arrive before they stopped serving Danishes at 10:30 A.M. After wolfing down a Danish and coffee, I was back at the club where I sneaked cookies and other sugary items until lunchtime. (In case of an "emergency," I always kept bags of Oreos or chocolate-chip cookies crammed in the glove compartment or stashed under the front seat of my car.)

For lunch I gave myself three options. First, I might bring a sandwich from home made with white bread, American cheese, and some sort of lunch meat smothered with mayonnaise which I ate with chips or potato salad. Sometimes I drove to the nearest salad bar where my plate quickly resembled a mountain of lettuce topped with heaps of grated cheese, crumbled hard-boiled eggs, sunflower seeds, croutons, macaroni salad, and two large ladles of Ranch dressing. But without question my preferred lunch was *fast-food drive-through bingeing.* Always alone, I'd drive up to McDonald's, Wendy's, or Dick's

Burgers (my local favorite) and buy two cheeseburgers with all the special sauces, two orders of large fries, and a large *Diet* Coke (you have to cut those calories anyplace you can!). Convincing myself I needed some fruit to balance out my meal, I'd also order an apple or cherry pie. Then off I drove with my big sack of food, which was always empty by the time I got back to work. If it was raining or if I was depressed, bored, or upset, I'd finish my McDonald's lunch, then drive right over to Wendy's where I'd repeat my entire order. At this point I was clearly eating "mood food"—that is, my food intake was directly related to my frame of mind. If anyone had discovered my unhealthy eating behavior back then, I'd have been devastated. After all, I was an aerobics instructor who preached a pretty good line about nutrition and health to her students. Little did they know . . . I was talking the talk, but I sure wasn't walking the walk.

Four o'clock in the afternoon always found me back at Dick's drive-up window asking for a *large* (these were *huge*) order of fries with the extra tartar sauce I preferred instead of ketchup. I guess I must have needed this extra "energy boost" before teaching my class at 5:00 P.M.—*right!*

Dinner wasn't nearly the production lunch was. Alone at night I mostly munched on finger foods or some kind of fast food I'd picked up on my way home from work—fish and chips, pizza, fried chicken, or more cheeseburgers. Then the TV went on, and I'd snack right up until bedtime. In the morning, the same old routine would start up again.

What was I thinking back then to have consistently ingested so much *garbage?* More accurately, what *wasn't* I thinking back then? No wonder I was having all kinds of physical problems—my poor system was just crying out for an overhaul! As I began counseling for my eating disorder and then as I began working with my personal trainer, it became clear that I was eating for just about every reason under the sun except that I was hungry. *I was living to eat, not eating to live.* If I ever expected to break my pattern of food abuse, I was going to have to take a long, hard look at my old eating habits and examine what food meant to me. In short, I was going to have to change the way I *thought* about food.

After months of hard work, my habits did change. Today I still eat a lot, I just eat *different* foods. For breakfast I'll usually have some of the following: whole-grain cereals with skim milk, fresh fruit, nonfat yogurt, omelettes made from egg whites and no cheese, whole-wheat bread with low-sugar jam, bagels with a touch of cream cheese (preferably nonfat), fruit juice, and potatoes pan fried with low-fat cooking spray.

More often than I like to admit, I eat lunch on the go—which usually means fast food. That's no excuse to drop the ball, however, and with a little creativity I find I have lots of healthy lunch options:

- A chicken-breast sandwich on a whole-wheat bun with lettuce and tomato (no mayonnaise—I'll add ketchup or BBQ sauce instead).
- A plain hamburger with lettuce, tomato, pickle relish, or ketchup.
- A baked potato with Light Ranch dressing and chives on the side (a healthier substitute for fries). (I might sprinkle on some Molly McButter or fat-free imitation bacon bits which I keep in my *large* purse. You wouldn't believe what I carry around in that thing; it looks like a condiment mini-bar!)
- A veggie burrito on a whole-wheat shell, or a veggie-and-chicken taco in a corn tortilla. (If cheese is an option, I'll order the light variety. I'll eat refried beans and Spanish rice, but I avoid *sour cream and guacamole*.)
- Chinese food orders include stir-fried chicken (without oil) or chicken skewers (grilled or broiled) and vegetable

dishes using as little oil as possible, *no* MSG, and steamed white rice.

- If I have a sandwich, I only order white meat (chicken or turkey) or tuna on whole-wheat bread with nonfat mayonnaise or Dijon-and-honey mustard. I try to avoid chicken, turkey, or tuna salad because they're usually loaded with mayonnaise.

My number-one choice for dinner is a combination of either chicken, fish, or extra-lean beef (only once a week), a green vegetable, and fruit. I love salads, and I make mine with unlimited amounts of lettuce and other fresh vegetables. If I'm at a restaurant salad bar, in addition to lettuce and fresh vegetables, I'll eat pasta (after draining the oil), egg whites, kidney and garbanzo beans, mushrooms, and *lite* croutons (I say No to the ones baked in butter), and use cheese and sunflower seeds only sparingly (although usually I pass them up entirely). I like shrimp and crabmeat, but they're high in salt so I make sure I'm drinking a lot of water when I use them in salads. As for salad dressing, I always go for the low-fat or fat-free varieties, or bring my own (another purse item) in a *small* container (not a huge sixteen-ounce bottle of fat-free Thousand Islands that causes customers to stop and stare). (A habit I've developed when eating salad is to pour the dressing on the side, then dip my fork into the dressing before I stab the lettuce and toppings. I save a lot of calories this way because a bare fork doesn't hold as much dressing as a chunk of lettuce does.)

Besides salads, I eat a lot of steamed vegetables like broccoli, cauliflower, peas, corn, squash, and zucchini. Baked potatoes covered with nonfat plain yogurt or nonfat sour cream with chives, Mrs. Dash light salt and pepper, or Molly McButter seasoning are also a favorite. Rice is always on my menu: brown rice, Spanish rice, and white rice with marinara sauce. I'll even eat pizza—yes, pizza—if it's made with part-skim mozzarella cheese, which I ask them to sprinkle on lightly, a light tomato sauce, fresh vegetables and fruit like mushrooms, green peppers, tomatoes, or pineapple. I avoid pepperoni, sausage, and other greasy meat toppings.

I will always have a sweet tooth, so for dessert I'll eat frozen non-fat yogurts, fat-free puddings, sorbets, sherbets, angel-food cake, fat-free cake (Entenmann's has a great selection of these), fat-free fruit newton cookies, or fresh fruit. Because I'm aware of the variety of healthy dessert alternatives available, now I can go through an entire holiday season without eating any chocolate candy! And let's face it, snacking is a part of life. Still, it doesn't have to be what causes me to lose my fight with fat. Between meals I munch on plain bagels, fresh fruit (apples, bananas, melon), nonfat yogurt, and rice cakes.

I love fruit juices, but I limit myself to two glasses when I'm counting calories. I also drink mineral water and limited amounts of diet sodas. Finally, I rarely go anywhere without my water bottle. I drink water all day long—at least eight to twelve 8-ounce glasses. (Not only is water an *essential* nutrient for your body, but it also plays a vital role in weight loss and weight-management programs.)

What a difference a change in eating habits can make! Today my engine runs smoothly and efficiently—you might even call it "turbo-charged." I have more energy, my total percentage of body fat is much lower, my health problems have cleared up, and my skin has a glow to it that it never had before. Getting from there to here wasn't easy, but I never gave up; I stuck to my "eating game plan," and over time I eventually replaced my old eating patterns with healthier, new ones. Food continues to be a major focus in my life, but it's a positive focus—one I can live with and accept. Deep down I know I'll never gain the weight again or resort to wild binges, but the fear that I might lose control is something that will always be there. For me, it's a mental challenge more than anything. Now let's look at how you can begin to gain control over *your* eating.

Step One: Change the Way You Think

I know not everyone has a problem with eating or with being drastically overweight, but most of us could stand to eat healthier, more nutritious foods. The fact is, studies continue to reveal not only that proper nutritional habits directly affect one's overall level of health, but they prove that maintaining a healthy diet actually helps *prevent* a multitude of serious illnesses as well. So *please* be clear about one thing: My message isn't "Get skinny," it's "Get fit and get healthy." And that means generating life-sustaining energy by eating healthier foods and exercising on a regular basis. In part three I'll talk more about exercise; right now I want to talk about what you're feeding that engine of yours, and *why*.

Ask yourself one simple question: Do you live to eat, or do you eat to live? If you eat to live, then you probably don't spend a whole lot of time thinking or worrying about food. Your nutritional program is fairly balanced (although you may slip up and splurge on chocolate occasionally), and all things considered you know there are more important things in life you'd rather be doing besides sitting around wondering what you'll have for dessert that night. To you, food is what it should be: fuel for your body. It is not a substitute for comfort or pleasure; eating is not something you do when you're depressed or angry. You enjoy food, but you certainly don't *live* for it. (On the other hand, if what you eat is *so low* on your list of priorities that you don't even give a second thought to what, when, or even *if* you consume, then that's something you need to become more aware of and change.)

If you're living to eat, however, food *is* a primary focus in your life—it consumes your thoughts and even your emotions (I used to think about what I was going to have for lunch while I was eating breakfast!). Meals are of utmost importance to you; you strategically plan each one as if you were planning a two-week vacation. This can be a dangerous relationship, one that can lead to eating disorders and eventually to numerous physical problems. You may not even know why or how you've developed this relationship with food. Your eating habits have been a part of you for so long that you've simply accepted them by now. Maybe you've even given up trying to change them.

Which best explains the role that food plays in your own life? *Are you eating to live, or living to eat?*

If you want to change your relationship with food and the control it has over you, first you must change the way you *think* about food. To help you do this, try remembering what events or situations in your past may have led you to your "live to eat" mind-set. Take a few minutes to answer the questions below.

1. Thinking back on your childhood, how important a role did food play in your life? What were you taught about food? Were you force-fed or made to clean every bite of food from your plate?

2. Some people eat to avoid unpleasant feelings; some people eat to prolong pleasant feelings. As a child, did you eat for reasons other than because you were hungry?

3. Can you see a relationship between the way you ate as a child and the way you eat today? If so, explain.

You may be having difficulty remembering some of these details, and that's okay. The point here is at least to get you to question and examine your former eating habits, the old ways of behaving that you may have unknowingly carried with you into the present. By doing this you'll discover some clues about your current eating patterns and behavior, plus gather some information which can help you begin to rethink the way you eat today.

Another effective way of helping you get a handle on why you eat the way you do is to keep a *food journal* for two to three weeks. I've always required my new clients to keep a food journal, and I've been keeping track of my food intake this way for over ten years. Start by purchasing a notebook small enough to fit in your purse or briefcase and carry it with you at all times. Below you'll see the basic food-journal format I've created with questions designed to make you think about and analyze your eating habits and behavior. Every day for the next two weeks, write down the following information:

- When you ate (the date and time)
- What you ate (be honest—everything counts!)
- Where you were when you ate (e.g., in the car, at your desk, standing outside)
- Why you ate/how you felt while you ate (e.g., you were hungry, you were bored, you were depressed)
- What you were doing while you ate (e.g., watching TV, reading the newspaper, walking around the kitchen)
- Whether you ate alone or with others

- What you did after you ate (e.g., continued sitting, took a nap, went for a walk, did the dishes)
- How you felt after eating (e.g., satisifed, stuffed, powerless)
- Any other thoughts related to food or your eating pattern that day (e.g., "The weather was crummy so I stayed inside and ate a doughnut instead of walking the dog"; "Yesterday I skipped dessert so I figured I deserved it today"; or "I was so excited I'd lost two pounds that I went out to lunch to celebrate!")

After two weeks you should have a fairly good picture of your current eating habits and patterns. What I often find with people who overeat (or eat in an unhealthy manner) is that some external event or circumstance always *triggers* an emotional reaction which in turn causes them to behave a certain way. A typical scenario might be knowing you're going to be late for work. This might cause you so much stress and anxiety that when you finally get to the office you react by raiding the employee kitchen and stuffing your face with Danishes. Intead of gobbling up doughnuts, however, you need to develop alternative plans of action; you need to begin channeling your energies in more positive directions when you feel those food triggers invading your brain. Don't reach for a doughnut; reach for a glass of water, then calmly go sit down at your desk. Instead of reaching for the cookie jar or cake plate when someone hurts your feelings, reach for your dance shoes, your walking shoes, or a good book (preferably *not* a cookbook!).

Reestablish your eating priorities and develop new strategies for gaining control over your eating. Set specific eating-related goals and determine specific actions like the following: "In two months' time I will no longer overeat whenever I feel depressed—instead, I will call my best friend or take a walk"; "Whenever I feel like eating a carton of my favorite ice cream, I will buy nonfat frozen yogurt or write in my journal instead" (This response is an effective one—once it took me *fifteen pages* before I overcame a particular food trigger, but in the end it really worked!); "I need to determine why I eat the way I do, so for the next three weeks I will keep a food journal which I will analyze regularly."

Changing the way you think about food involves changing behavior patterns (and old internal tapes) that you've been carrying around with you for most of your life, and that's not easy. There are no absolutes; there isn't *one way* that works. Examining my past and keeping a food journal helped me question and eventually change the way I thought about food, and it's worked for many of my clients as well. Not only that, keeping a food journal is easy and doesn't cost more than the price of a small notebook (a lot less expensive than therapy!). But in the end you must develop your own personal system for coping with your feelings and creating positive, new alternatives for old behavior patterns. Make a commitment to yourself and *get going.* If I could do it, so can you!

▼

Think long-term, but take action now! The results are up to you.

Chapter Four:
Choosing the Best Fuel

Nutrition 101

Nutrition science can be a highly complicated subject, but you don't have to devote long hours to the subject to absorb its fundamental principles. If you don't already know the basics of good nutrition, now's the time to learn.

At the simplest level, food is fuel for your body—it supplies your body with the energy you need to function on a daily basis, it enables your body to repair and grow new tissue, and it regulates your metabolic functions. Food is broken down into chemical components called *nutrients*. There are six classes of nutrients: water, minerals, vitamins, carbohydrates, proteins, and fats.

WATER   The most essential of all the nutrients is water. Water makes up 60 percent of your body weight, and it's necessary for energy production, for temperature control, and for the elimination of waste products from your metabolic system. If you make only one dietary change as a result of this book, make it an increase in your daily water intake, especially if you suffer from water retention. Most women don't drink enough water, and that sends a signal to their bodies to hold on to what little water they have (just as starvation dieting sends the signal to hold on to "precious" fat). One of the best ways to relieve water retention is by drinking more water. Suddenly your metabolic system has what it needs; it relinquishes the rest and cleanses your body in the process. *Drink at least eight 8-ounce glasses of water a day.*

MINERALS   Chemical processes in your body demand various minerals for their successful completion. Minerals such as calcium, phosphorus, and zinc are an integral part of bones, teeth, blood, and nerve cells. Another mineral, iron, is an essential component of hemoglobin and necessary for the formation of red blood corpuscles, and also a component of certain respiratory enzymes.

VITAMINS   In order to maintain good health you need certain vitamins in your diet. Vitamins play an important role in a complex series of chemical reactions that convert fat and carbohydrates to energy; they also assist in bone and tissue formation, growth and repair, and function as metabolic regulators. There are two kinds of vitamin classifications: water soluble and fat soluble. Water-soluble vitamins, like B-complex and vitamin C, are not stored in your body and must be ingested daily. Fat-soluble vitamins are those stored in body fat (primarily the liver) and include vitamins A, D, E, and K. Consuming more fat-soluble vitamins than your body needs over long periods of time can produce toxic effects. *Eating a balanced diet almost always takes care of your vitamin and mineral requirements, but if you feel that these needs aren't being met, consult a dietician or physician.*

CARBOHYDRATES   These are the most readily available source of food energy. During the digestion process, all carbohydrates are broken down into simple sugar glucose and become the body's primary energy source. There are two kinds of carbohydrates: complex and simple (or refined). Complex carbohydrates supply important nutrients and fiber needed to regulate your system and can be found in whole grains, pasta, beans, fruits, and vegetables. Simple carbohydrates found in sugar and other sweets represent an energy source but have no other nutritional value. *Think (and eat) complex, not simple.*

PROTEINS   Proteins build and repair body tissue and form enzymes, hormones, red blood cells, and antibodies. Proteins in both plant and animal sources are composed of amino acids, and of the twenty amino acids, nine are essential to good health. Foods such as milk, cheese, eggs, fish, poultry, and red meat are called complete proteins because they contain all nine essential amino acids. Complex carbohydrates such as grains, beans, and vegetables are incomplete proteins because they do not contain all of the nine amino acids. However, when you combine certain incomplete proteins, like rice and beans, they bring together the necessary amino acids and form complete proteins. *In my opinion, protein has gotten a bum rap in recent years. Americans do not eat "too much protein," as we're often told; we eat too much fat. Cut your fat intake first, then worry about the protein.*

FATS   Fats (also called lipids) are the most concentrated source of food energy. They insulate and protect the body's organs against trauma and exposure to cold, plus they're involved in the absorption and transport of fat-soluble vitamins. Fats are also the source of fatty acids, which are divided into two categories: saturated and unsaturated (which includes polyunsaturated and monounsaturated fatty acids). Saturated fats (ones that harden at room temperature) are found in certain meats, dairy products, and plant oils and are the least desirable of all fats because they build up on the walls of your arteries and tend to raise your blood cholesterol level. On the other hand, polyunsaturated fats, like those found in some vegetable and fish oils, are fine in moderation. *You need some fat in your diet, but that's no excuse for having it hang over your belt, okay?*

The healthiest, most effective eating program is one that includes the proper amount of the six essential nutrients as found in the four foods groups: Dairy, Meats, Fruits and Vegetables, and Grains and Cereals. Recently, the U.S. Department of Agriculture revealed new findings regarding the ideal American diet in the shape of a food-guide pyramid. According to the USDA's pyramid chart, our daily food intake should include the following:

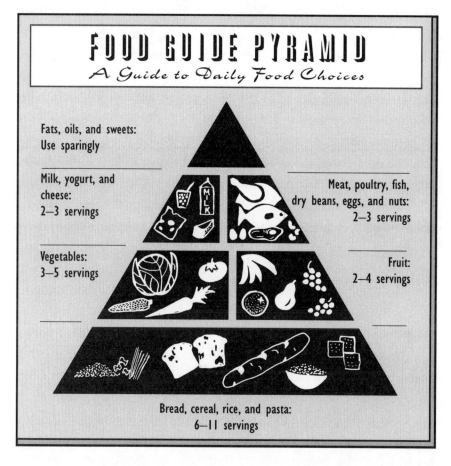

FOOD GUIDE PYRAMID
A Guide to Daily Food Choices

Fats, oils, and sweets: Use sparingly

Milk, yogurt, and cheese: 2–3 servings

Meat, poultry, fish, dry beans, eggs, and nuts: 2–3 servings

Vegetables: 3–5 servings

Fruit: 2–4 servings

Bread, cereal, rice, and pasta: 6–11 servings

Although your daily intake may vary slightly (for example, if you're involved in a weight-loss program, have strict dietary requirements due to certain medical conditions, or are involved in rigorous athletic training), on the whole this is a guide that you should look to when you're making your daily food choices.

Fat Facts

No matter what they say, no matter what you tell yourself, there are no miracle diets, no overnight cures, no revolutionary concepts. Good health and a lean body come from knowledge, patience, and discipline. If you want to lose weight and eliminate your excess body fat, you'll have to eat more nutritious foods, reduce the fat in your diet, and exercise regularly. That's all there is to it.

After taking countless courses in nutrition and trying just about every weight-loss program in the country, I'd simply *had it* with overweight diet counselors and chain-smoking physicians telling me how to permanently lose weight and get fit. Although I still had not attained my personal weight-loss goals, I began thinking about how I might help others reach similar goals of their own. Combining my knowledge of nutrition and weight loss with my professional training in aerobics and fitness, I formed my own company to counsel on weight loss and weight management and to do body-composition analyses and fitness counseling. My goal was to help average people discover nutrition and fitness programs that worked for their particular life-styles, and for several years I offered encouraging words to others but seldom took the time to motivate myself or heed my own advice. When I started working with my trainer, Davis, however, I began taking more a of personal interest in the information that I was dispensing and eventually was able to incorporate it into my own life. Because of this newfound confidence in myself and pride in my accomplishments, my business began to thrive. In one year alone I tested 2,000 clients to determine their body compositions—their lean body mass and fat mass percentages. (To date, my company has tested approximately 20,000 clients, and that number continues to grow.)

If there's one thing I've learned through my years of weight-loss

▼

In the beginning there was muscle . . . now there's a lot of fat.

and weight-management counseling, it's that *bodies don't lie*. If you eat right, exercise, manage stress effectively, and make a concerted effort to enjoy life and give to others, your entire being will reflect that. But one of the first steps toward achieving a healthy, fit body is to determine what you're made of: you need to have a body-fat analysis done.

Already I can hear some of you asking yourself, "Why would I want to *pay* someone to give me a test that would tell me *exactly* how fat I am? I already *know* how fat I am—I can see *that* from looking in the mirror and reading the numbers on my bathroom scale." Okay, so you already know that your clothes are too tight and maybe you're about twenty pounds heavier than you'd like to be, but do you know how much of that weight is fat and how much is lean body mass? Your bathroom scale is not an accurate measure of your *total body composition*—vital information to have before successfully embarking on any weight-loss or fitness program. Your scale at home just shows you why you can't zip up your jeans anymore. The kind of weight you want to lose is *fat*, not lean body mass, and unless you know how much of it you have, how will you know how much of it you need to lose? If you don't know your starting point, your *total body composition*, I guarantee you'll be on a diet roller coaster for the rest of your life. Let me explain. . . .

Lean Body Mass Versus Fat Mass

First, your total weight is composed of two things: lean body mass and fat body mass. Your lean body mass is the active part of your body, the *live* part of you, the engine that makes you run—your muscles, bones, and blood. Your lean body mass supports your skeletal system, it dictates your posture—and, most important, it determines your health and how you function on a daily basis. Your lean body mass requires a certain amount of fuel to operate: nutrients from food and water, plus oxygen. Operating a bit like a furnace, it burns carbohydrates for quick energy and relies on fat reserves for lengthy, sustained aerobic activities like brisk walking, jogging, or aerobic dance. The more lean body mass you have, the more heat and energy your engine generates; thus, the more effective your metabolism and the more calories you burn. Your healthy future depends on the amount of lean body mass that you have, and you can increase it with proper exercise and a sound nutritional program.

Whatever does not qualify as lean body mass is fat. There are three kinds of fat in your body: *essential fat*, which pads your internal organs and is necessary for health; *intramuscular fat* situated between your muscles; and *subcutaneous fat*, visible fat (What you see is what you ate!) located beneath the skin on top of the muscle. I like to think of subcutaneous fat as "fat that won't fit on the inside." Unlike lean body mass, fat is *inactive*; it is simply the stored, unused energy from the calories that you consume. If you consume more calories than your lean body mass can burn up, guess what? It turns to fat. *Although some amount of fat in your body is essential, in general the less of it you have the healthier you'll be. Too much body fat is dangerous: Heart disease, the number one killer in America, has been directly linked to poor nutritional habits and obesity.*

Body Composition Analysis

The type of analysis (or test, as it's also called) that my company uses to discover clients' body composition is called Bioelectrical Impedance, or B.E.I. B.E.I. uses a computer with an impedance meter to measure the amount of fat versus lean body mass in a person's body. Attached to the computer are two wire cables with metal teeth at the ends. These teeth hold small pads which a technician affixes to designated areas of the right wrist and foot. After personal data such as height, weight, activity level, and age are entered into the computer, the meter is turned on and it sends a small, undetectable electrical current through the body to calculate the following information: total percentage of body fat, total fat weight, total lean body mass weight, suggested ideal weight, and estimated basal metabolism (the calories a person should consume based on his/her *total lean body mass*). (Remember, the lean body mass requires the fuel and energy; the fat mass requires no active maintenance.) The more lean body mass a person has, the faster the current travels. This is because muscle tissue from the lean body mass is 70 percent water—an excellent conductor of electricity. The more fat in a person's body, the slower the current will travel; the fat *impedes* the current.

There are other methods used for analyzing body composition, such as hydrostatic weighing, ultrasound, calipers, and girth measurements. There is one thing to keep in mind, however: No method is 100 percent accurate. Short of dying and having your fat surgically removed and then measured, the key is to find a convenient method that you can have performed on a regular basis (every three to four months until you reach your goal, then once yearly thereafter) and to find a technician you trust. The best place to have your body composition analyzed is at a reputable health club, a sports-medicine clinic, or by a registered dietician, chiropractor, or physician. Check the yellow pages in your phone book for leads, then call to find out who gives body-composition analyses and what kind of method they use. Also try to determine how long they've been doing the tests and ask for references so that you can verify their credibility and the accuracy of their methods. Currently, a standard body-composition analysis costs between $10 to $20.

Here are two examples of one of my clients' Body Composition Profiles using the Bioelectrical Impedance method. The first shows a body-fat percentage of 28.5, a fat weight of 42.7 pounds, and a lean body mass weight of 107.3 pounds. The second, conducted approximately three and a half months later, after "Jane Doe" followed the initial weight-loss recommendations, shows a body-fat percentage that has been reduced to 22.9, a fat weight of 30.7 pounds, and a lean body mass of 103.3 pounds. Jane has cause to celebrate!

Experts don't necessarily agree on the recommended range for lean body mass weight and total body-fat percentage for men and women. However, the clients I've tested who've demonstrated the most success in terms of improving their overall health and level of physical fitness have fallen somewhere within the following ranges:

LEAN BODY MASS WEIGHT

(Remember: This chart does not depict total target weights, only lean body mass target weights, which you can only obtain by having a body-fat analysis.)

▲ WOMEN		▲ MEN	
4'10"	80–88 lbs.	5'4"	105–120 lbs.
5'0"	85–95 lbs.	5'6"	110–130 lbs.
5'2"	92–97 lbs.	5'8"	118–140 lbs.
5'4"	97–102 lbs.	5'10"	128–160 lbs.
5'6"	102–107 lbs.	6'0"	139–175 lbs.
5'8"	105–111 lbs.	6'2"	145–182 lbs.
5'10"	107–115 lbs.	6'4"	151–191 lbs.
6'0"	112–120 lbs.	6'6"	160–200 lbs.

The ideal percentage of body fat for women is 18 to 22 percent; for men it's 10 to 14 percent. These numbers are not absolute, however—they're simply a gauge and represent an approximate goal to achieve (having slightly more or less lean body mass or body fat than what these figures suggest is all right). *Remember: The quantity of your lean body mass helps to determine the quality of your health.*

BODY COMPOSITION PROFILE

Date: 09/26/91

Jane Doe

Time: 15:35:23

Sex: *Female*
Height: *65.00 in.*

Step test score: *N/A*
Resistance: *520 ohms*

Age: *37*
Weight: *150.00 pounds*

Activity level: *Moderate activity*
Reactance: *56 ohms*

Percent Fat: 28.5%

The normal range of body fat for a 37-year-old female is *21.0 to 27.0%*, with an average of *25.0%*. You are above the expected value.

Fat Weight: 42.7 pounds

This is your total fat expressed in pounds. The normal range of fat weight for a female of your age and weight is from *31.5 to 40.5 pounds.*

Based on your data: This is too much fat! You need to reduce your body's weight by at least *14.2 pounds*. For more information, see weight-loss recommendations.

Lean Body Mass: 107.3 pounds

Your lean-to-fat ratio is *2.51* and can be used as a convenient index of your body composition. It should be your goal to make your lean-to-fat ratio as high as possible. A value of *3.00* or higher would be desirable for you. You can increase your lean-to-fat ratio by engaging in vigorous exercise, especially circuit weight training. You have approximately *35.1 liters* of total body water, or *51.6%* of your body weight.

Recommendations for Jane Doe

Your initial target weight is 131.8 to 139.8 pounds.
This weight range will normalize your body's fat content compared with others of your sex and age. As your body weight decreases, an exercise and nutrition program will decrease the amount of lean body mass lost. Remember, it's your body's content of excess fat that you should be concerned about.

Weight-Loss Recommendations

Based on your lean body mass and current activity level, your estimated basal metabolism is *1598 Kcal*. In order to lose weight at a safe and consistent level, it is recommended that you have a net intake of approximately *1,289 calories per day*. At this caloric level you will lose weight at a rate of approximately *1.4 pounds* per week.

In most cases, weight loss includes the loss of fat and lean body mass. In order to reduce the amount of lean body mass lost, it is recommended that *you exercise at least 3 days per week* (preferably more). Only with a dietary/exercise program will it be possible to reach your goal weight of *135.8 pounds* in *71 days*, with as little loss of muscle as possible. Below is your personalized weight-loss chart, which shows your rate of weight loss and when you will reach your recommended body weight.

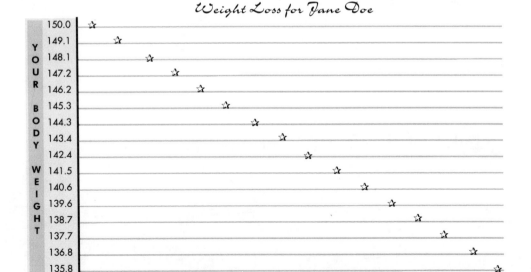

Weight Loss for Jane Doe

YOUR BODY WEIGHT

150.0
149.1
148.1
147.2
146.2
145.3
144.3
143.4
142.4
141.5
140.6
139.6
138.7
137.7
136.8
135.8

0   5   9   14   19   24   28   33   38   43   47   52   57   61   66   71

DAYS TO REACH GOAL WEIGHT

Exercise Recommendations

Different types of aerobic exercises should be done at least *3 days per week*, a minimum of *20 minutes per session*, and at a minimum intensity level of *60 to 80 percent of your maximum heart rate.* In your case, your training heart-rate zone would be *110 to 146* beats per minute. Regular exercise will promote optimal body composition (decreased fat and increased lean mass). The table below lists the calories that you will expend depending on how much time you exercise.

Exercise	*Time in Minutes*								
	10	20	30	40	50	60	80	90	120
WALKING (15–17 MIN./MILE)	54	109	163	218	272	327	435	490	653
JOGGING (10–12 MIN./MILE)	112	223	335	446	558	670	893	1004	1339
RUNNING (9 MIN./MILE)	131	263	394	525	657	788	1051	1182	1576
SWIMMING (CONTINUOUS CRAWL)	106	212	318	425	531	637	849	955	1274
CYCLING (9.4 M.P.H.)	68	136	204	272	340	408	544	612	816
BASKETBALL	94	188	282	376	469	563	751	845	1127
RACQUETBALL	119	238	357	476	595	714	953	1072	1429
GARDENING	63	126	188	251	314	377	502	565	754
NAUTILUS CIRCUIT	61	122	183	244	305	366	488	549	732
UNIVERSAL CIRCUIT	79	158	237	316	395	474	632	711	948
FREE WEIGHTS CIRCUIT	58	116	174	232	290	348	464	522	696
AEROBICS (CONTINUOUS)	116	231	347	463	578	694	925	1041	1388
TENNIS (CONTINUOUS)	74	148	222	297	371	445	593	667	890
GOLF (CARRYING BAG)	58	116	174	231	289	347	463	521	694

THIS OR ANY OTHER EXERCISE/NUTRITION PROGRAM SHOULD NOT BE UNDERTAKEN WITHOUT THE ADVICE OF YOUR HEALTH-CARE PROFESSIONAL.

(Calories Expended Based on Your Weight)

BODY COMPOSITION PROFILE

AFTER PROFILE

Date: 01/13/92   *Jane Doe*   **Time:** 15:40:18

Sex: *Female*
Height: *65.00 in.*

Step test score: *N/A*
Resistance: *510 ohms*

Age: *37*
Weight: *134.00 pounds*

Activity level: *Moderate activity*
Reactance: *65 ohms*

Percent Fat: 22.9%

The normal range of body fat for a 37-year-old female is *21.0 to 27.0%*, with an average of *25.0%*. You are less than the expected value.

Fat Weight: 30.7 pounds

This is your total fat expressed in pounds. The normal range of fat weight for a female of your age and weight is from *28.1 to 36.2 pounds*.

Based on your data: Your body fat is within the normal range for a female of your age and weight. However, you may wish to further increase your lean body mass and decrease your body fat content. This can be done by maintaining an active exercise program while paying close attention to good nutritional practices.

Lean Body Mass: 103.3 pounds

Your lean-to-fat ratio is *3.37*, and can be used as a convenient index of your body composition. It should be your goal to make your lean-to-fat ratio as high as possible. A value of *3.00* or higher would be desirable for you. You can increase your lean-to-fat ratio by engaging in vigorous exercise, especially circuit weight training. You have approximately *34.4 liters* of total body water, or *56.7%* of your body weight.

Recommendations for Jane Doe

Your optimal weight is 132.0 to 138.0 pounds. This weight range places you within the normal limits of body fat for a female of your age. By following an exercise program you can further reduce your fat content and increase your lean body mass.

Congratulations

Your body weight and fat are within normal limits for your age and sex. Keep up the good work. Your predicted basal metabolism based on lean body mass is *1,554 calories* per day.

Exercise Recommendations

Different types of aerobic exercises should be done at least *3 days per week*, a minimum of *20 minutes per session*, and at a minimum intensity level of *60 to 80 percent of your maximum heart rate*. In your case, your training heart rate zone would be *110 to 146 beats per minute*. Regular exercise will promote optimal body composition (decreased fat and increased lean mass). The table below lists the calories that you will expend depending on how much time you exercise.

Exercise	*Time in Minutes*								
	10	20	30	40	50	60	80	90	120
WALKING (15–17 MIN./MILE)	49	97	146	195	243	292	389	438	584
JOGGING (10–12 MIN./MILE)	100	199	299	399	498	598	797	897	1196
RUNNING (9 MIN./MILE)	117	235	352	469	587	704	938	1056	1408
SWIMMING (CONTINUOUS CRAWL)	95	190	284	379	474	569	759	853	1138
CYCLING (9.4 M.P.H.)	61	122	182	243	304	365	486	547	729
BASKETBALL	84	168	252	336	419	503	671	755	1007
RACQUETBALL	106	213	319	425	532	638	851	957	1276
GARDENING	56	112	168	224	281	337	449	505	673
NAUTILUS CIRCUIT	55	109	164	218	273	327	436	491	654
UNIVERSAL CIRCUIT	71	141	212	282	353	423	565	635	847
FREE WEIGHTS CIRCUIT	52	104	156	207	259	311	415	467	622
AEROBICS (CONTINUOUS)	103	207	310	413	517	620	827	930	1240
TENNIS (CONTINUOUS)	66	133	199	265	331	398	530	596	795
GOLF (CARRYING BAG)	52	103	155	207	258	310	413	465	620

THIS OR ANY OTHER EXERCISE/NUTRITION PROGRAM SHOULD NOT BE UNDERTAKEN WITHOUT THE ADVICE OF YOUR HEALTH-CARE PROFESSIONAL.

(Calories Expended Based on Your Weight)

Cutting Your Intake

The typical dieter's weight is like a yo-yo: it goes down for a few days or a few weeks, then it comes right back up again. The bathroom scale becomes the enemy; what it reads can make or break a dieter's day. But the critical issue with weight loss is not *how many* pounds are lost, but *what kind* of pounds and *how many inches* are lost. That's why it's so important to have a body-composition analysis done if you're considering beginning a weight-loss program. *Again, only through body-composition analysis can you learn how to set the healthiest, most effective weight-loss goal for yourself: a proper balance between your lean body mass and your fat mass.*

There is a way (*really*, there is) to achieve that goal, but there are also countless other carefully crafted marketing ploys all promising that their products will give you a permanently thin, lean body—and in only one week! Don't be fooled; they don't work. *I* should know.

There's also the old "when-all-else-fails method" to losing weight: self-starvation. Unless you become hooked on this method (and you can—it's called anorexia nervosa), it won't work either. In fact, in the long run you'll be doing yourself more harm than good. When you continuously cut calories below a healthy recommended level, your total body composition changes. Most of the initial weight that you lose is water, and if you're not exercising you will also lose muscle. Unfortunately, fat is usually the last thing to disappear. (Also, the older you are, the less able your body is to replace vital lost tissue.) This kind of yo-yoing puts tremendous stress on the body's system. Medical scientists have found that rapid weight loss dramatically alters the body's metabolic rate and its calorie-burning efficiency. When you eat normally your body's metabolic function increases to stimulate the digestive process, which in turn utilizes more calories by producing heat and energy. But when you go on severely restrictive diets, this process slows down. Your body perceives that it's actually starving and tries to preserve all the energy it can by turning down its thermostat, thereby reducing the rate at which calories are burned. Starving actually makes you *fatter*, because it's those fat energy reserves that your body begins rebuilding at a faster rate—hardly the result you were after.

I know I've said it before, but here it is again: *The best way to lose weight safely and permanently is to eat a balanced diet, one that's low in fat and low in total calories, and to exercise regularly.* Having read Nutrition 101, you already know what constitutes a balanced diet. Now you need to know how to determine the number of calories that it's safe for you to consume whether your goal is to lose weight, maintain your weight, or increase your weight.

It takes approximately 15 calories per pound of body weight per day to maintain your current weight. Therefore, if you weigh 140 pounds, you need 2,100 calories daily to remain at 140 pounds. If you want to lose 10 pounds, then obviously you must consume fewer calories and/or increase your activity level. The American Medical Association recommends that you lose no more than about 2 pounds per week (much more than 2 wouldn't be effective in the long run). Don't ever cut your daily intake below a reasonable amount: for women that's about 1,200 calories; for men, about 1,500–1,800.

You know how to lose weight by cutting calories, but in order to lose the *kind* of weight that you want to, namely the fat pounds, simple calorie cutting won't work. You're going to have to do something about preserving those lean body mass pounds (specifically the muscles) that increase your metabolic rate and burn your fat calories instead of stashing them away on your thighs or around your hips. The less muscle you have, the less you can eat—and in order to build muscle, you're going to have to *exercise*.

Sometimes people will complain to me that after weeks of watching what they eat and exercising regularly they still *weigh* the same (even though their clothes fit better or are actually looser). Unfortunately, they're still measuring their success only by what that bathroom scale tells them. As a way of explaining to them why they still weigh the same despite obvious improvements in their health and physique, I cite the following example. Let's say we took two overweight women and put them on a diet consisting of 1,200 calories per day. One woman was told to exercise regularly, the other was told not to exercise at all. After seven weeks on the program, the woman who did not exercise lost eighteen pounds (twelve total inches): eleven pounds of fat and seven pounds of lean body mass. The woman who exercised lost twenty-three pounds of fat, but at the same time gained four pounds of lean body mass, which led to an overall weight loss of nineteen pounds (sixteen total inches)—only one pound less than the nonexerciser. The woman who exercised clearly ended up with the best overall results, but she won't know that unless she follows up her program with a body-composition analysis to see precisely what kind of weight she lost and what kind of weight she gained. (And later, if both women regain the weight that they lost initially, the nonexercising woman will quickly gain back a larger percentage of body fat, plus her metabolism will have been reduced so that any future weight loss will take place at a much slower rate.)

Not only is the body composition of the exercising dieter different (healthier) than the nonexercising dieter, she also has lost inches from her waistline, hips, and thighs by replacing fat with muscle. Contrary to popular opinion, muscle does not weigh more than fat. Muscle is simply denser and more concentrated than fat. In fact, one pound of fat takes up to three times more space (on your body) than one pound of muscle. It weighs the same, but the fat is *triple* the volume—it fills up those jeans at three times the speed of muscle! I have tried to lose weight by simply cutting calories and by cutting calories and increasing my activity level, and I'll tell you this: I would *never* consider dieting without exercising. After all, what good is it to lose twenty pounds and still have flabby, mushy, jiggling buns? You can finally fit those buns into your blue jeans, but who's going to want to squeeze them?

An Attitude to Eat and Live By

When you're dieting, stop worrying about the wrong foods and start looking for the right ones. Don't waste time and energy thinking about what you *can't* have; instead, focus on what you *can* have. So many people associate dieting and changing their eating habits with deprivation, pain, and loss—loss of comfort, flavor, fun, spontaneity, social eating, ice cream, candy . . . That doesn't have to be the case. Replace the word *diet* with *eating plan* or *eating program*, and see if some of the negative connotations and feelings disappear. Begin viewing your "diet" as a healthy, organized, and well-thought-out way of eating. There are many flavorful, fun, low-fat food choices out there. Begin thinking about the wonderful things you're doing for your body and the wonderful things you'll get in return, not the least of which are improved health, renewed energy, and enthusiasm for life. Your engine needs good fuel, not garbage—you wouldn't put it into your car's engine, so stop putting it into your body's.

One final piece of advice about dieting: Beware of certain friends when you're trying to change the way you eat. They may really love you, but they're not always the best support systems at times like these, particularly if they're not dieting themselves. I can still hear some of mine, in fact: "C'mon now, *girlfriend*, it's just one little piece of pie. It's not going to *kill* you. Go ahead, I won't tell anyone you ate it. . . ." Ha! She won't have to *tell* anyone—everyone will *see* that piece of pie all over my hips! Surround yourself with positive, inspirational people—ones who recognize the value of the goals you're shooting for and who will support (not sabotage) you along the way.

Savvy Shopping

Because grocery shopping is the prelude to eating healthy foods at home, you want to make sure that your cupboards and refrigerator are stocked with foods that work *for* you, not *against* you. First, some grocery shopping ground rules:

1. *Always shop with a prepared list.* How many times have you made up your list then promptly left the house without it? Stick to your list; it'll keep you from succumbing to "bargains" that you can easily live without. (Forget the price—do you really *need* thirty packages of Top Ramen noodles? They're over 50 percent fat!)

2. *Never grocery-shop when you're hungry—everything looks good!* If you eat before going shopping, not only will you be less likely to buy things you don't need, but you'll also be less tempted to taste-test all the mouth-watering samples offered to you on a toothpick by smiling Jimmy Dean Sausages marketing representatives.

3. *Know your budget.* Shopping on payday can be dangerously expensive because you always feel somewhat richer on this day. If you don't believe me, compare payday shopping bills with those of a few days earlier. When the cash flow is slower, you'll usually make smarter purchases.

4. *Don't take an "aisle vacation."* Going down every aisle in the store usually isn't necessary and often leads to a grocery cart loaded with junk. Stay away from the aisles that contain hard-to-resist munchies and sweets such as cakes, pies, cookies, candies, and chips.

Be selective about where you shop for your groceries. Everywhere you turn you'll see "Super Grocery Stores" that are long enough to hold a 10K race. If you're like me, you're often so exhausted by the time you even *get* to the grocery store at the end of the day that you simply aren't up to sprinting down twenty-five different aisles in search of dinner. It takes forever just to find anything in these stores, plus at the end of the first aisle your cart is usually half full of items that serve absolutely no purpose but that somehow *looked* appealing. Always shop at the same grocery store, and if you can, go there during off-hours—you'll already know where everything is located, you'll avoid long lines, and you'll be less tempted by the king-sized Snickers bars surrounding the checkout counter while you're waiting to pay.

Next, get a "fat-finder's license"; that is, learn how to recognize foods that contain a lot of fat (or any other ingredients that you want to avoid like sugar, salt, preservatives) and substitute those foods for ones that contain less fat. *Look beyond the attractive marketing claims on the outside of packages and begin reading the nutritional labels. Terms like "light," "l-i-g-h-t," "lite," or "l-i-t-e" don't always mean the food is low (light) in fat.* Nutritional labels contain a lot of important information; however, since some of it can be confusing, you'll need to learn how to decipher that information.

The first thing you'll usually see on a nutritional label is the serving size and the number of servings per container, followed by a number representing calories, and below that a nutrient breakdown list (e.g., protein, fat, carbohydrates). The nutrients are derived from the ingredient list, which is often given last, and those ingredients are always listed in this order: primary ingredient, secondary ingredient, and so on. For example, if an ingredient list reads rolled oats, brown sugar, rice, sunflower oil, etc., that means the food item contains more rolled oats than anything else, next brown sugar, and on down the list. Let's stop here: Although nutrition labels give you total calories in a serving of food, they don't always break down the number of grams of nutrients into calories. (In fact, by law manufacturers are only required to list nutrients by weight, not by percentage of calories.) And as a bona-fide fat finder, you need to know what percentage of the total calories is in each gram of protein, carbohydrates, and fat.

The following sample of nutrients and their calories per gram are universal and cannot be questioned:

NUTRIENT	CALORIES PER GRAM
Protein	4
Carbohydrates	4
Alcohol	7
Fat	9
Water	0

Once you know these numbers, all you have to do is a little multiplication with the numbers on your food labels to determine total calories per gram. For example, here's a label from a typical bag of potato chips:

NUTRITIONAL INFORMATION PER SERVING

Serving size: 1 ounce
Servings per container: 15
Calories [per serving]: 150
Protein [per serving]: 2 grams
Carbohydrates [per serving]: 18 grams
Fat [per serving]: 8 grams

Using the fixed nutrient/calories-per-gram chart above, let's take the numbers from the bag of chips and determine what percentage of calories come from each specific nutrient:

Protein: 2 grams (from chip label) x 4 (from fixed chart) = 8 calories.

Carbohydrates: 18 (from chip label) x 4 (from fixed chart) = 72 calories.

Fat: 8 (from chip label) x 9 (from fixed chart) = 72 calories.

Now here's how the chips convert onto this new chart:

NUTRIENT	CALORIES	CALORIES/SERVING	TOTAL CALORIES
Protein	8 calories	divided by 150 x 100 =	5.3%
Carbohydrates	72 calories	divided by 150 x 100 =	48%
Fat	72 calories	divided by 150 x 100 =	48%

As you can see, almost 50 percent of the calories from one serving of these potato chips come from fat. If you're trying to eat foods that derive 30 percent (or less) of their calories from fat, these chips exceed your allotted fat intake by 20 percent. So, put them back on the shelf right now! Using the fixed chart to convert the nutritional numbers from your food labels will help clarify what the labels are *really* saying. Although the pretty packaging may promise "90 percent fat free," your own calculations will reveal an entirely different story; what you see isn't necessarily what you're getting. Beware of those hidden enemies! (A good rule of thumb is that there should not be more than three grams of fat per 100 calories. This would make the product 30 percent fat, which is the maximum percentage of fat that you should consume if you're trying to lose weight and body fat.) No, you don't have to wear a calculator around your neck to survive in this confusing world of label mumbo jumbo. You'll need to do the math at first, but eventually you'll be able to quickly determine what it is that you need to know about the food you're purchasing.

Thus far I've been talking primarily about deciphering nutritional labels for fat content. However, there are other ingredients that you should be on the lookout for, one of which is sodium (salt). Too much sodium can lead to high blood pressure, hypertension, and severe water retention. The maximum recommended amount per day of sodium is 2,400 milligrams. Be sure to read your labels, particularly

▼

Two scoops of ice cream contain more fat than 4,700 cups of zucchini. Try fitting that on your sugar cone!

on inherently salty foods such as pickles, olives, canned goods, chips, and lunch meats.

Now let's take a quick trip down the aisles together, and I'll give you a few more tips about shopping. . . .

FROZEN FOODS

Buy: Plain frozen vegetables are fine; so are many of the frozen meals available today. Thanks to the avant-garde thinking of certain food manufacturers, you can now purchase frozen meals that are low in fat, calories, cholesterol, and sodium. Try to keep your selections (per serving) below 320 calories, with 5 to 10 grams of fat (2 grams of saturated fat) and 750 milligrams of sodium. Add a whole-grain dinner roll and a small tossed salad and *voilà!* Dinner in no time!

Don't buy: Frozen vegetables laden with cream and cheese sauces contain a lot of fat, sometimes as much as 25 grams—*Ugh!* Also avoid pot pies, macaroni-and-cheeses dishes, and heavily breaded foods like fish and chicken. Read the labels on TV dinners and frozen kids' meals—some have more than 5 grams of fat per serving.

Remember: If you must make a decision between canned or frozen vegetables, go with the frozen ones because they usually contain less salt, preservatives, and additives.

DAIRY PRODUCTS

Buy: You can purchase cheese products with little to no fat, but often the sodium content is high. Try to keep your cheese fat content between two to five grams. Always choose skim or low-fat milk or 2 percent milk (you'll be saving yourself about three or four grams of fat this way), and look for fat-free, low-fat, or nonfat versions of other staple dairy items like margarine, cream cheese, cottage cheese, and sour cream. There are also many dairy desserts to choose from—nonfat frozen yogurts, ice milks, sherbets, and puddings. (But be careful not to load them up with nuts and other sweet, fattening toppings. Try topping them with fresh fruit instead.) Eggs are eggs; not much can be done to alter their content, so watch your consumption of these—three with yolks should be all you need per week. (When I cook, I usually use only the egg whites, because it's the yolk that contains all the cholesterol and fat.)

Don't buy: Limit your intake of regular cheese and avoid whole milk, cream, butter, sour cream, cream cheese, and cottage cheese.

Remember: Almost every dairy product has a low-fat or nonfat equivalent these days, so buy the healthier versions—your arteries will thank you.

MEATS

Buy: Look closely at your meats and read the labels (for example, there's a *big difference* between how manufacturers prepare whole, fresh turkeys—compare them!). If there's a lot of visible fat, ask your butcher to trim it or select another cut. (Why pay for something that you're going to throw away?) With any meat purchase, the key words to look for are *lean, extra-lean,* or *low fat,* particularly with beef and pork purchases. Try these low-fat versions of your old standbys: low-fat hot dogs, Canadian or imitation bacon, turkey or chicken sausage. White meat from poultry is preferable to dark meat because it contains less fat. Some types of fish have a higher fat content than others, but white fish such as halibut, cod, pollack, and red snapper are always safe bets. Crab, lobster, and shrimp are good seafood choices. Always buy tuna packed in water, not oil.

Don't buy: Most regular canned meats, packaged luncheon meats, hot dogs, sausage, and bacon are loaded with fat, so read your labels carefully. Chances are you'll begin avoiding these items altogether.

Remember: Keep your intake of red meat to a minimum: Two 6 ounce servings (no more) is all you really need per week. Here's a low-fat meat-buying guide that I think you'll find helpful:

LOW-FAT MEAT-BUYING GUIDE

▲ POULTRY

Chicken
Turkey
Cornish game hens
Quail

▲ FISH (FRESH OR FROZEN)

Bass	Perch
Bluegill	Pike
Catfish	Pollack
Cod	Sea Trout
Croaker	Shark
Flounder	Smelt
Greenland Turbot	Snapper
Grouper	Sole
Haddock	Walleye
Halibut	Whiting

▲ SHELLFISH (FRESH OR FROZEN)

Oysters	Lobster
Clams	Scallops
Crabmeat	Frogs' legs

▲ BEEF —
RECOMMENDED CUTS
Roasts:

arm
chuck (round bone)
rump
sirloin tip
eye of round

Steaks:	flank
	round
	tenderloin
	sirloin tip
Misc.:	extra lean ground beef
	lean stew meat
	ground beef — round
	ground chuck

▲ PORK	loin chops
	pork tenderloin
	boiled sliced ham*
	center ham slice*

▲ LAMB	leg of lamb or loin roast
	leg chop steak
	rib, shoulder, sirloin, and leg chops
	shanks
	arm chop

▲ VEAL	veal cutlet
	loin chop
	rib chop
	blade steak
	rump and sirloin roast

Contains more than 100 mg. sodium per serving

PRODUCE

Buy: Virtually all fresh fruits and vegetables are terrific, so eat up!

Don't buy: There are a few hidden culprits in the produce section. Limit your purchase of avocados, nuts, and oil-marinated vegetables.

Remember: It's the preparation of vegetables and fruits that can get you into trouble. *Eat raw or lightly steamed produce items. Don't fry them in heavy oils, butter, or add a lot of sugar. No cream or cheese sauces, either.*

BREADS AND CEREALS

Buy: Whole-grain products are healthier, so read your labels to make sure that the first ingredients listed in your breads and rolls are whole grains—corn, oats, bran, rye, etc. Also make sure that the sugar, salt, and fat contents are low. Buy pita bread, bagels, low-fat or fat-free muffins, cakes, and pastries, fat-free crackers or saltines.

Don't buy: Items that list "enriched" flour as one of the first ingredients are telling you that the most prevalent ingredient has been stripped of its natural fiber and other important nutrients, which are then synthetically replaced (that's what "enriched" means), so don't buy them. High-fat breads and rolls include: croissants, biscuits, scones, doughnuts, and Danishes. Many breakfast cereals contain huge amounts of sugar (particularly commercial granolas), so flip the box over and decide for yourself if you're making a wise purchase or not.

Remember: Don't be fooled by brown-colored bread bags or bread that's been colored brown by molasses or other coloring. *Read your labels.*

MISCELLANEOUS ITEMS

▲ SOUPS AND CANNED GOODS *Buy:* Low-salt and low-fat soups, sauces, and vegetables are the ones to buy; however, don't necessarily trust the front label. Check the back panel to confirm the claim.

Don't buy: Many canned goods contain high levels of salt (sodium). If you're watching your salt intake, buy the low salt variety or choose a frozen equivalent.

▲ SALAD DRESSINGS *Buy:* Look for dressings that contain no more than two grams of fat per tablespoon (fat free). Again, don't trust your selection just because the bottle claims to be "lite"—use your fat finder's know-how and read the label carefully.

Don't buy: You can cancel out all your good intentions concerning fresh vegetables and fruit salads by dumping high-fat dressings on top (regular mayonnaise is a big no-no). Buy only those that are fat free or low in fat.

▲ DESSERTS *Buy:* Fat-free cookies and cakes are terrific tasting and readily available. Also, head back to the dairy and/or frozen-food sections for nonfat and sugar-free frozen yogurts, ice milks, puddings, fat-free dessert bars, and Jell-O.

Don't buy: Regular cookies, cakes, pies, ice cream, and puddings contain tons of fat and sugar. Stop and ask yourself, "Is it worth it?" *If you don't buy it, you won't eat it.*

▲ MUNCHIE SNACKS *Buy:* Your labels can tell you the types of oils and preservatives used, plus the fat content, and there are actually a lot more healthier snack choices these days than you might think: pretzels, fat-free tortilla chips, oyster crackers, rice crackers (spiced and flavored), graham crackers, vanilla wafers, bagels, light popcorn (no butter), and fruit-based cookies, just to name a few. (Don't forget those fresh fruits and vegetables, too!)

A word about snacking: Because I suggest that you not go for more than four hours without eating something, snacking between meals is inevitable. The key to smart, controlled snacking (versus panic snacking) is to be prepared by having healthy snacks (like the ones listed above) on hand. Keep them in your car or your purse, at your desk at work or in your cupboards at home. Don't starve yourself. When you need quick refueling, go for it—just make healthy choices.

Don't buy: Do I really have to tell you who these guys are?

Somehow they just have a way of ending up in your cart, don't they? Mixed nuts, potato chips, corn chips, candy bars, cookies, buttered popcorn . . . Oh, *please*—put the stuff back on the shelf and head for the produce section ASAP!

There you have it—enough pointers to turn you into a permanently savvy shopper. Once you start putting them into practice, you'll be amazed at the difference a few small changes can make: *Your healthier food purchases won't put a strain on your budget, plus they will make you feel better, give you more energy, and help you control your weight, too.*

Health-Conscious Cooking

Cooking in a healthier, fat-free mode has a lot to do with awareness and adaptation. Small changes in your cooking habits can cut down on your total caloric, fat, sugar, and salt intake and add more fiber and other beneficial nutrients. Just because a recipe calls for a half cup of *butter* and a cup of *whole milk*, for instance, doesn't mean you can't substitute other, less fattening ingredients. Recipe cards aren't etched in stone. Whatever kinds of food you prepare, from soul food to Chinese, Mexican, or Italian, with a little imagination, experimentation, and creativity, you can modify many of your recipes and cooking methods to make healthier, more nutritious meals—and still retain the original flavor.

Let me show you what I mean by ingredient substitution using a few simple recipes below. (The total calories listed are for the *entire recipe*, not individual servings.)

(ORIGINAL RECIPE)

Boil in salted water:

2 cups macaroni

Drain. Return it to the saucepan.

Over low heat stir in:

1/2 cup light cream

Put the macaroni in a dish and sprinkle with:

1/2 cup or more of grated cheddar cheese

Total calories: 898

Total fat calories: 443.61 (49.29 grams of fat)

Macaroni
and
Cheese
(4–6 Servings)

Now here's the same recipe after changing certain ingredients:

(MODIFIED VERSION)

Boil in water:

2 cups macaroni

Drain. Return it to the saucepan.

Over low heat stir in:

1/2 cup skim milk

Put the macaroni in a dish and sprinkle with:

1/2 cup or more of grated low-fat cheddar
cheese

Total calories: 442.9

Total fat calories: 9 (1 gram of fat)

Tacos

(3–6 Servings)

(ORIGINAL RECIPE)

Sauté until golden brown:

　　1 finely chopped onion

in:

　　2 tablespoons butter

Add and simmer for 3 minutes:

　　$1/2$ cup tomato juice

　　1 cup cooked ground beef or ground pork
　　　　sausage

　　$1/8$ teaspoon thyme

　　1 teaspoon salt

Set this filling mixture aside, then fry in deep
　　fat heated to 380° until golden:

　　6 tortillas

Remove from the fat and drain. Fill with meat
　　mixture. Top with grated cheese, avocado,
　　and sour cream.

Total calories: 1,483.5

Total fat calories: 891.36 (99.04 grams of fat)

Look at the difference simple substitution can make:

(MODIFIED VERSION)

Sauté until golden brown:

　　1 cup finely chopped onion

in:

no-stick skillet or 3 teaspoons corn oil

Add and simmer for 3 minutes:

$^1/_2$ cup tomato juice

1 cup shredded cooked chicken (skin
removed)

$^1/_8$ teaspoon thyme

1 teaspoon lite salt, Mrs. Dash seasoning

Set this filling aside, then lightly fry in corn
oil heated to 380° until golden:

6 tortillas

Remove from oil and drain. Fill with meat
mixture. Top with grated low-fat cheese,
low-fat yogurt, low-fat sour cream, or
low-fat cottage cheese, and fresh diced
tomatoes.

Total calories: 877.5
Total fat calories: 272 (30.3 grams of fat)

(ORIGINAL RECIPE)

Preheat oven to 425°.

Grease muffin tin with butter, oil, or bacon
drippings. Place it in the oven until sizzling
hot. Sift together:

$^3/_4$ cup sifted all-purpose flour

2 $^1/_2$ teaspoons double-acting baking pow-
der

2 tablespoons sugar

1 teaspoon salt

Corn Bread Muffins

*(about fifteen
2-inch muffins)*

Add:

> 1 1/4 cups yellow or white stone-ground cornmeal

Beat in a separate bowl:

> 1 egg

Beat into it:

> 3 tablespoons melted butter or bacon drippings
>
> 1 cup milk

Combine all ingredients with a few rapid strokes. Place the batter in the hot muffin tin. Bake corn bread for 25 minutes.

Total calories: 821
Total fat calories: 424.3 (52.7 grams of fat)

(MODIFIED VERSION)

Preheat oven to 425°.

Spray muffin tin with Pam cooking spray.

> Place it in the oven until sizzling hot. Sift together:
>
> > 3/4 cup sifted all-purpose flour
> >
> > 2 1/2 teaspoons double-acting baking powder
> >
> > 1 tablespoon artificial sweetener
> >
> > 1/8 teaspoon lite salt

Add:

> 1 1/4 cups yellow or white stone-ground cornmeal

Beat in a separate bowl:

    1 egg white

Beat into it:

    3 teaspoons corn oil

    1 cup skim milk

Combine all ingredients with a few rapid strokes. Place the batter in the hot muffin tin. Bake corn bread for 25 minutes.

Total calories: 585

Total fat calories: 173. 7 (19.3 grams of fat)

See how easy that is and see the amount of calories and fat you can eliminate? Take a look at your favorite recipes and try experimenting with ingredient substitution. Here's a sample list of substitutions to consider:

▲ INSTEAD OF:	▲ USE:
oil	water, corn oil
whole milk, cream	skim milk
sour cream, cream cheese	low-fat or nonfat yogurt and cottage cheese, low-fat sour cream, nonfat cream cheese
butter	low-fat margarine
eggs	more egg whites, fewer egg yolks
cheese	low-fat or nonfat cheese
ice cream	ice milk, nonfat frozen yogurt
mayonnaise	low-fat yogurt mixed with buttermilk
salt	herbs and spices, lite salt

refined flour	whole-wheat flour
sugar and honey	apple or pineapple juice
beef stock	vegetable stock, chicken stock with fat removed
ketchup	homemade tomato sauce
canned vegetables	fresh vegetables

Not only can you improve your recipes through ingredient substitution, but other simple changes in the way you *prepare* and *cook* your foods can save a lot of unnecessary calories and fat, too. Next time you're considering popping those pieces of chicken in the frying pan, consider the following alternatives:

▲ INSTEAD OF:	▲ TRY:
frying or deep frying	baking, broiling, or grilling
leaving fat and skin on meats	removing *all* of the fat and skin
coating food in bread crumbs	experiment with other spices

Become a health conscious cook: Substitute for high-fat ingredients ones that have a lower fat content, and eliminate cooking methods that add unnecessary fat to your foods and strip them of essential nutrients.

Fast Fill-ups

Unless you live on a sunny, tropical island where the hours glide by unnoticed while you lounge on the beach casually nibbling fresh pineapple, papaya, and grilled mahimahi, chances are your life more closely resembles the noisy, fast-paced atmosphere of the Indy 500: Up at 6:00 A.M., you rush around all day at top speed tending to your children, your spouse, your job, your home, your pets, and your shopping, eating whatever candy bar is handy and making pit stops at the closest fast-food restaurant for just enough fuel to keep you going until the race is over and the crowds have all gone home to bed. *Whew!* Welcome to life in the '90s. . . .

Your busy life-style will probably never ease up until you move to that villa in the Caribbean, but that's no reason to ignore your body by feeding it garbage fuel and then expect it to give record-breaking performances every day. Sooner or later your engine will sputter, lose its momentum, and simply break down. You can forget about *winning* the race; you probably won't even *finish* it. Now is the time to start paying more attention to your body and to the food that you feed it. As with much of what you do in life, the key to consuming nutritious fuel is: (1) know the outcome that you want; (2) plan ahead; and (3) make smart choices. Here are some suggestions on how to incorporate healthy eating into your hectic life-style of fast food and restaurant dining.

Breakfast

As soon as you get up in the morning, *eat something.* People tell me all the time, "If I eat breakfast I'll be hungry all day long!" Well, guess what? You're *supposed* to feel hungry every few hours or so—that's your body's way of telling you it needs nutrients. Get your metabolism going with fresh fruit, a plain bagel, a fat-free muffin, oatmeal, or whole-grain cereal with skim milk. If you regularly eat breakfast from a bag (that is, from a fast-food restaurant), steer clear of high-fat and high-sodium items like egg sandwiches, sausage, ham, croissants, biscuits, and deep-fried french-toast sticks. Do order muffins or pancakes, and use a little jam instead of butter. Watch your caffeine consumption, too. In fact, why not try decaffeinated for a change?

Lunch

Back at Burger King again? Okay, but hold on: Most burgers, fish fillets, chicken sandwiches, and fries are loaded with as much fat and sodium as you require for the *entire day*. Pull out your fat finder's license and examine the choices before you order. These are just a few *safe fast foods* to consider at lunchtime:

- Char-broiled chicken sandwiches without mayonnaise
- Garden salads with fat-free dressing (Don't you have that in your purse someplace?)
- Baked potato with lite Ranch dressing or imitation sour cream
- Chicken burrito with lettuce and tomato (no cheese, sour cream, or guacamole)
- Small hamburger with a little ketchup or mustard only, lettuce and tomato
- Pizza made with light cheese, light sauce, and vegetable topping (or none at all—it's not bad, really!)

Remember to stick with regular-sized portions—no double McFats, please—and drink either skim milk or water instead of soda pop or milk shakes.

You can also make your job easier by asking for a nutritional listing of the items that your fast-food restaurant serves. Most will have this information available, but if not write to the Center for Science in the Public Interest (CSPI) in Washington, D.C., and ask for a copy of their fast-food eating guide.

Dinner

You've successfully navigated your way through breakfast and lunch, and now it's dinnertime. A word of warning beforehand: If you usually eat dinner much later than 7:00 P.M., remember that your metabolism is just about ready to call it quits by then. Whether you prepare dinner at home, bring dinner home, or eat dinner out, the best foods to eat are ones that are low in fat, salt, and simple carbohydrates and high in protein and complex carbohydrates. Protein is necessary for muscular growth and repair—something that your body does while you sleep at night. Your body uses nutrients from carbohydrates for physical and mental energy, so you're better off eating your carbohydrates during the day. Don't make your system work overtime during the night with unwanted carbohydrates and fats—it will cost you, believe me.

Restaurant dining presents special challenges for the health-conscious eater. You see so many tempting choices on the menu that sometimes it's hard to control yourself. Before heading out to dinner, mentally plan what you might order: broiled fish, baked chicken without the skin, pasta prepared with a light sauce, a plain baked potato, salad with dressing on the side. Still, don't deprive yourself, either. After all, if you're out to have good time and you see something on the menu that you simply can't live without, go ahead and order it—but then eat only half of what's on your plate. Share the other half with your dinner companion or take the remaining portion home to be eaten *tomorrow* (not later that night!).

Also, watch out for menu lingo (those semi-sophisticated terms that you seldom use to refer to your own cooking at home). Don't be afraid to ask what something means, how something's prepared, or to say how you'd *like* it prepared. For example, "Alfredo," "Mousseline," "Newburg," "Bearnaise," and "Hollandaise" all basically mean the same thing: sauces with a lot of egg yolks, butter, and/or cream. If the menu says something is crispy, deep fried, pan fried, or sautéed, don't order it. Instead, go for steamed, poached, broiled, or grilled, and make sure it's not basted with fat during cooking.

The "power meal" isn't really a fat steak, a baked potato covered with butter and sour cream, or a chef's salad swimming in Roquefort dressing. *You* have the power—the power to say No and choose items from the menu that benefit your body and your health. And if you do occasionally overdo it, don't panic—just get back on the track as soon as you can. It takes 3,500 calories to put on a pound of fat, and you probably didn't eat *that* much. Take a look at why you overate, and next time avoid the same scenario by planning your dining-out strategy ahead of time.

Finally, if your eating is driven by social activities, maybe it's time to cut back on the number of times you eat out, or change your social activities to more active ones like roller-blading, tennis, racquetball; or weight lifting. Skip the "Happy Hours." Personally, I don't see how inhaling a pile of fattening hors d'oeuvres and watered-down drinks can make you happy anyway. A more appropriate name might be "Unhappy Hour." If you must attend these functions because of your job, eat a healthy snack beforehand so you won't be as tempted by greasy tidbits, and limit your alcohol to one drink (go for lite beer if it's available). Better yet, drink club soda or tonic with lime, or just plain water. Make your own "Happy Hour" by doing things you enjoy and devoting time to your own personal improvement, or by sharing your time with others: Take an aerobics class, browse through your favorite bookstore, play with your children, or take them to the park.

Whatever your solution for sane social eating, recognize your weaknesses but remain in charge and in control. *Anticipate the hairpin turns and stay in the driver's seat!*

Lean-Machine Maintenance

Eating healthy, nutritious foods is so simple. Once you know about basic nutrition and how your body uses the fuel that you give it, you can begin making a lifetime habit of choosing better foods for yourself and for your family. Great new products fill your grocery-store shelves, and terrific books about food, nutrition, and healthy eating continue to flood the marketplace every year. I have only touched the surface with the information in chapters 3 and 4, so don't stop learning about these very important topics. *When you stop learning, you stop growing.*

I can't come home with you every night and help you fix dinner, and I can't whisper, "Stop—don't eat those!" into your ear as you reach for another handful of potato chips. What I can do is remind you once more to consciously and carefully consider every food choice that you make throughout your day. I can ask you to think about what your health and your life really mean: Are you willing to risk not seeing your children grow up or your grandchildren graduate from college? Do you want to live long enough to finally step off your Indy 500 fast track, relax, and enjoy your retirement? Don't eat for how you look today; eat for how you'll feel tomorrow, and the next day, and the day after that. Life is beautiful—look outside, take a walk, feel the freedom and embrace the experiences and challenges that come your way. Learn to love yourself the way you deserve to: The greater self-love, the less food love. *Set yourself up to win and go for it!*

A Diet Plan for Maximum Fat Loss

Throughout this book I've emphasized the importance of setting goals for yourself, taking control of your life, and *taking action*. If one of the goals of your nutrition and weight-management program is to lose unwanted body fat, I'm making your job a lot easier by giving you the specific eating plan that I've followed for years and that I recommend to my clients as well. This plan came about as a result of several things. First, as a bodybuilder, I needed to devise a nutritional program that would allow me to obtain maximum muscle definition—one that would increase my lean body mass and decrease my body fat. Second, as a woman who loved food, I knew I'd never stick with a program that required me to starve myself. Whatever program I devised had to include a variety of balanced foods that I could consume frequently (and without guilt) throughout the day. Third, since I traveled a great deal, the program had to be simple, flexible, and include foods that were easily accessible. The plan that I developed successfully accomplishes all three. It will work for you, too.

Beginning on the next pages you'll find a chart depicting daily serving recommendations from each of the four food groups (plus a miscellaneous group that includes things like margarine, oil, coffee creamer, etc.) for the women's 1,200-calorie plan and the men's 1,500-calorie plan. These plans are set up for *sedentary, nonactive* individuals—those people who do not get much physical exercise beyond their day-to-day office or at-home jobs. Active individuals, those who exercise regularly or whose daily jobs require strenuous physical activity, can increase the total calories to 1,500 (women) or to 1,800–2,000 (men). Following this chart, I've given you a list of specific foods to eat and shown what constitutes one serving from each group. *I recommend that you remove these pages from the book (or photocopy them), tape them to your refrigerator, or carry them with you in your briefcase or purse. Better yet, stick them inside that new food journal of yours and you'll have them right at your fingertips all day long.*

FIRST, SOME GUIDELINES TO FOLLOW:

1. Before beginning this or any eating-related program, you should obtain your physician's approval.
2. Eat every three to four hours.
3. Drink eight to twelve 8-ounce glasses of water daily.
4. Use the foods suggested as a *foundation*. You can devise a more personal plan based on your food preferences and your life-style; however, pay close attention to the amount of fat in the foods that you choose and don't add any extra fat through food preparation—keep your foods as close to their natural states as possible. (To ensure weight loss, women should not consume more than thirty

grams of fat per day; men shouldn't consume more than forty grams of fat per day. You may want to purchase a fat-gram counter to help you make the best low-fat choices.)

5. *Balance* is the key to this eating plan. If you don't quite eat the exact number of servings recommended, that's okay—just don't go overboard with one food group and ignore the others.

6. Don't *exceed* the serving sizes. Just as adding fat to this plan will defeat its overall effectiveness, so will eating much more than the portions suggested.

7. Eat the majority of your food before 5:00 P.M., when you're most active. (When you eat and then immediately go to sleep, your fat cells celebrate by partying all over your hips and thighs!)

8. Don't drink more than two cups of coffee per day, and/or two diet sodas.

▲ FOOD GROUP	▲ 1,200 CALORIES DAILY	▲ 1,500 CALORIES DAILY
1) Bread, cereal, rice, & pasta	4 servings	5 servings
2) Vegetable & fruit	5 servings	6 servings
3) Milk, yogurt, & cheese	4 servings	4 servings
4) Meat, poultry, fish, & beans	3 servings	3 servings
5) Other (oils, margarine, coffee creamer, etc.)	2 servings	3 servings

Bread, Cereal, Rice, and Pasta

(This group includes whole-grain breads and whole-grain cereals that have low sugar content. Nutrients include: carbohydrates, fiber, and roughage.)

ONE SERVING =

1 medium slice whole-grain bread
2 small slices diet bread
1 small dinner roll
1 pita pocket bread
$^1/_2$ bagel
$^1/_2$ oz. fat-free cake
2 fat-free cookies
2 graham crackers
6 saltine crackers
2 cups cooked lite popcorn

$^1/_2$ cup cooked: rice, cereal, pasta
1 4-inch pancake
1 homemade low-fat muffin
1 small piece corn bread
1 tortilla shell; 1 oz. no-oil tortilla chips
2 rice cakes
1 cup whole-grain cereal (cold)

Vegetables and Fruit

(This group includes predominantly green and yellow vegetables, plus all fruits. Nutrients include: vitamins, minerals, carbohydrates, and fiber, also a high percentage of water.)

ONE SERVING =

Fruit:
1 medium-sized orange, pear, apple, peach, nectarine
$^1/_2$ mango
$^1/_2$ banana
2 plums
$^3/_4$ cup raspberries, blueberries
$^1/_2$ cup pineapple, grapes,
1 cup strawberries, melon
$^1/_4$ cantaloupe

4 dates

$^1/_2$ cup lite canned fruit

$^1/_2$ cup real fruit juice (not fruit drinks)

Vegetables:

2 cups lettuce

1 cup raw or cooked asparagus, bamboo shoots, broccoli, brussel sprouts, green beans/peas, cabbage, carrots, celery, cauliflower, collard/mustard greens, mushrooms, spinach, squash (all kinds), sauerkraut

$^1/_2$ cup corn

1 large cucumber, tomato

$^1/_2$ baked potato, $^1/_2$ baked yam

Milk, Yogurt, and Cheese

(This group includes skim milk, low-fat cheeses, cottage cheese, ice milk, and nonfat yogurts. Nutrients include: vitamins A and D, calcium, minerals, and protein.)

ONE SERVING =

1 cup skim milk

1 oz. cheddar, provolone, mozzarella, American cheese

2 slices fat-free cheese

$^1/_2$ cup low-fat cottage cheese

1 cup nonfat yogurt

1 cup fat-free pudding

3 oz. nonfat frozen yogurt

1 tbsp. imitation sour cream

Meat, Poultry, Fish, and Beans

(This group includes lean and extra-lean meats, cuts that are low in fat content. Nutrients include: protein and iron.)

ONE SERVING =

(Remove all fat and skin before eating.)

3 oz. extra-lean beef

3 oz. chicken (dark meat)

3 oz. lean pork

3 oz. salmon

3 oz. water-packed canned tuna

4 oz. cod, halibut, or other white fish

4 oz. shrimp

4 oz. turkey or chicken (white meat)

6 egg whites

$1/2$ cup cooked: black beans, black-eyed peas, kidney beans, garbanzo beans, lentils, lima beans, northern/navy beans, pinto beans

Other

(This group includes condiments and other additives used to enhance or change food flavor. Most condiments are unnecessary; however, it may take some time to readjust your palate and begin eliminating your favorite high-fat ones. Nutrients include: negligible.)

ONE SERVING =

1 tsp. margarine

2 tsp. low-fat margarine

1 tsp. oil

1 tsp. regular salad dressing

2 tbsp. fat-free salad dressing

1 tbsp. lite Cool Whip

1 tbsp. light coffee creamer

1 tbsp. nonfat mayonnaise

4 tbsp. low-sugar jam

2 tbsp. Molly McButter

2 oz. tomato sauce—e.g., spaghetti, pizza sauces

Here's a sample of what you could eat in a week's time on my diet plan based on approximately 1,200 calories per day and using the foods listed above:

BREAKFAST (7:00 A.M.)

> 1 cup cooked oatmeal
>
> $1/2$ cup skim milk
>
> 1 peach
>
> 12 oz. water

SNACK (10:00 A.M.)

> 1 cup nonfat Jell-O pudding
>
> $1/2$ cup grapes
>
> 12 oz. water

LUNCH (12:30 P.M.)

> 1 sandwich (2 slices diet bread, 3 oz. tuna, 1 tbsp. nonfat mayonnaise, 3 leaves lettuce, 2 slices tomato)
>
> 1 oz. no-oil tortilla chips
>
> 12 oz. water

SNACK (3:30 P.M.)

> 1 cup strawberries (optional: 1 tsp. light Cool Whip topping)
>
> 12 oz. water

DINNER (6:30 P.M.)

> 1 chicken breast (baked or broiled)
>
> 1 large green salad (3 cups total) with 2 tbsp. nonfat salad dressing

Day One

$^1/_2$ baked potato with 2 tbsp. Molly McButter

3 oz. nonfat frozen yogurt

12 oz. water

SNACK (9:00 P.M.)

1 slice fat-free cheese

$^1/_2$ apple

8 oz. water

*Optional daily: 2 cups coffee, tea, and/or 2 diet sodas

BREAKFAST (7:00 A.M.)

1 cup whole-grain cereal

$^3/_4$ cup skim milk

$^1/_2$ banana

$^1/_2$ cup fruit juice

12 oz. water

Day Two

SNACK (10:00 A.M.)

1 apple

6 saltine crackers

$^1/_2$ cup skim milk

12 oz. water

LUNCH (12:30 P.M.)

1 medium green salad with diced chicken (white meat) and 2
   tbsp. nonfat salad dressing

1 medium baked potato with 1 tbsp. imitation sour cream, 2
   tbsp. Molly McButter

4 oz. nonfat frozen yogurt

12 oz. water

SNACK (3:30 P.M.)

1 low-fat bran muffin

$^1/_2$ cup fruit juice

12 oz. water

DINNER (6:30 P.M.)

4 oz. white fish (baked or broiled)

1 cup cooked green vegetables

$1/2$ cup brown rice (with nonfat topping)

1 whole-grain roll

12 oz. water

SNACK (9:00 P.M.)

1 cup Jell-O fat-free pudding

8 oz. water

Day Three

BREAKFAST (7:00 A.M.)

2 slices diet whole-wheat toast with 4 tsp. low-sugar jam

4 egg whites (hard-boiled)

1 cup strawberries and melon

1 cup skim milk

12 oz. water

SNACK (10:00 A.M.)

1 apple

12 oz. water

LUNCH (12:30 P.M.)

1 medium hamburger patty (optional: lettuce, tomato, pickle, ketchup, mustard)

1 small green salad with 1 tbsp. nonfat salad dressing

1 pear

12 oz. water

SNACK (3:30 P.M.)

$1/2$ toasted bagel (optional: 2 tsp. low-sugar jam)

12 carrot sticks

12 oz. water

DINNER (6:30 P.M.)

   1 cup cooked pasta with 2 oz. tomato sauce

   $1/2$ oz. grated nonfat cheese topping

   1 slice whole-grain bread

   1 cup cooked green and yellow vegetables

   12 oz. water

SNACK (9:00 P.M.)

   3 oz. nonfat frozen yogurt with fresh-fruit topping

   8 oz. water

Day Four

BREAKFAST (7:00 A.M.)

   1 cup nonfat fruit yogurt (sprinkle in $1/2$ cup whole-grain cold
      cereal)

   1 slice diet bread

   1 orange

   12 oz. water

SNACK (10:00 A.M.)

   $1/8$ slice melon

   1 slice diet bread with 1 tsp. low-sugar jam

   12 oz. water

LUNCH (12:30 P.M.)

   1 chicken burrito (with lettuce, tomato, and onions—*no gua-
      camole, cheese, or sour cream*)

   1 small green salad with 1 tbsp. nonfat salad dressing

   1 oz. no-oil tortilla chips with 2 oz. salsa

   12 oz. water

SNACK (3:30 P.M.)

   8 carrot sticks; 8 celery sticks; 8 cucumber slices—dip in nonfat
      Ranch dressing

1/2 apple

12 oz. water

DINNER (6:30 P.M.)

1 medium turkey-breast patty

1 medium green salad with 2 tbsp. nonfat salad dressing

1 whole-grain dinner roll

2 cups sugar-free Jell-O

12 oz. water

SNACK (9:00 P.M.)

1 cup fresh strawberries with 1 tbsp. lite Cool Whip

8 oz. water

BREAKFAST (7:00 A.M.)

1 4-inch pancake with 1 cup fresh berries

1 cup nonfat yogurt

12 oz. water

SNACK (10:30 A.M.)

1 bran muffin with 2 tsp. low-sugar jam

12 carrot sticks

12 oz. water

LUNCH (12:30 P.M.)

1 large bowl homemade navy bean soup

1 medium green salad with nonfat salad dressing

1 peach or nectarine

12 oz. water

SNACK (3:30 P.M.)

1/2 banana

1 rice cracker

12 oz. water

Day Five

DINNER (6:30 P.M.)

    4 oz. cod (baked or broiled)

    1 cup cooked mixed vegetables

    $^1/_2$ cup white rice with marinara sauce

    12 oz. water

SNACK (9:00 P.M.)

    1 oz. fat-free pound cake topped with $^1/_2$ cup fresh berries and 1
       tbsp. lite Cool Whip

    1 cup hot tea (decaffeinated)

Day Six

BREAKFAST (7:00 A.M.)

    1 cup hot cereal with 1 cup skim milk

    1 orange

    12 oz. water

SNACK (10:30 A.M.)

    2 slices fat-free cheese

    1 cup fresh vegetables (carrots, cauliflower, broccoli, etc.)

    12 oz. water

LUNCH (12:30 P.M.)

    1 sandwich (2 slices diet bread, 3 oz. white turkey meat, lettuce,
       tomato, Dijon mustard, and/or nonfat mayonnaise)

    1 oz. no-oil tortilla chips

    1 peach

    12 oz. water

SNACK (3:30 P.M.)

    2 fat-free cookies

    1 cup skim milk or fruit juice

    12 oz. water

DINNER (6:30 P.M.)

Red beans and rice (1 cup beans, $^1/_2$ cup white rice)

1 medium piece corn bread

1 cup cooked green vegetables

12 oz. water

SNACK (9:00 P.M.)

1 oz. fat-free cake

1 cup hot peppermint tea

BREAKFAST (7:00 A.M.)

1 omelette made from 4 egg whites and 1 yolk, 1 cup chopped

vegetables, 2 slices nonfat cheese

1 slice diet toast with 1 tsp. low-sugar jam

1 cup fresh fruit

12 oz. water

Day Seven

SNACK (10:30 A.M.)

$^1/_4$ melon

2 graham crackers

12 oz. water

LUNCH (12:30 P.M.)

1 large bowl homemade black bean soup

1 whole grain roll

1 medium green salad with nonfat salad dressing

1 plum

12 oz. water

SNACK (3:30 P.M.)

1 cup raw vegetables dipped in 2 tbsp. nonfat salad dressing

$^1/_2$ banana

12 oz. water

DINNER (6:30 P.M.)

   4 oz. turkey breast

   $1/2$ cup mashed potatoes with 1 tsp. low-fat margarine

   1 cup cooked carrots and broccoli

   2 fat-free cookies

   12 oz. water

SNACK (9:00 P.M.)

   $1/4$ melon

   2 cups cooked lite popcorn

   8 oz. water

Remember, to make this eating plan work, to increase muscle definition and replace unwanted body fat with lean body mass, you'll also need to *exercise*. Now it's on to part three to develop a personalized workout program. Are you ready? Let's *move it!*

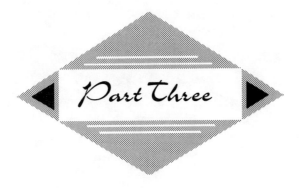

Part Three

MOVE IT!

Your body is your home; if you don't maintain it,
where will you live?

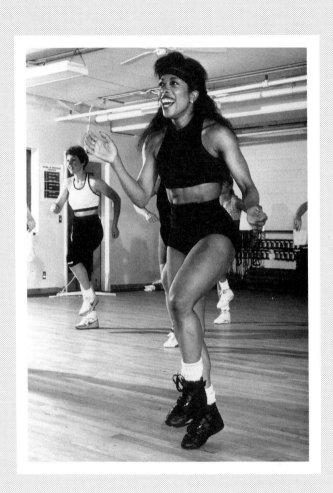

Chapter Five:
Motion Stimulates Emotion

Think about this: How does your body perform when you're sad, feeling hopeless, or depressed? You walk slowly and your shoulders are slumped, your breathing is quiet (except for the occasional loud *sigh*), and your face looks hollow and drawn. On the other hand, when you're happy, motivated, or excited, you walk faster, your heart beats more rapidly, your breathing is quick, and your eyes are open wide—your whole body is *alive*. People can tell how you're feeling just by watching you. Your body language sends signals to others: It either welcomes them or warns them to stay away. *Next time you're feeling down and depressed, change the way you're moving and you'll change the way you feel!* If you're sitting down, get up! Stand up and stand tall! Take deep, controlled breaths and begin stimulating your nervous system. Take a brisk walk, run up the stairs as fast as you can, turn up the stereo and dance around the living room. Once you start moving, an amazing transformation takes place: All the negative emotions you were feeling begin to disappear, and soon they're replaced by positive, empowering emotions. *Motion stimulates emotion: Use physical activity to lift your spirits and create the positive results you want.*

When you're born, no one gives your parents a neatly packaged owner's manual containing operating instructions or troubleshooting or maintenance tips. It is their job to give you a solid foundation for living, which includes instilling in you values and giving you the tools necessary for personal growth and development. And if your parents were like mine, they did the best job they could—probably using many of the tools *their* parents gave them. When we're young, we seldom question our parents' teachings, but by the time we're adults we've usually developed our own road maps for living which are a combination of our parents' lessons and lessons we've learned through our own personal experiences. While I was growing up, exercise and physical activity (other than work in the fields) was not something my family participated in. My own life experiences, however, have taught me that exercise is a *necessary*, not an *accessory* part of life training. *Without physical energy it's difficult to have mental energy: You can't separate the two.*

If one of the goals you wrote down earlier in this book includes beginning a regular exercise program (and I hope it is!), then before you do one stretch, before you put your foot on a step or pick up a single barbell, first ask yourself, "Why am I doing this?" Do you plan to work out so that when bikini season rolls around you won't be ashamed to put yours on? Do you plan to lift weights in order to develop the hard body of your dreams? Although you need these kinds of short-term goals to keep you motivated, I've got some news for you: If you are *only* working out to drop some weight or shape up your body, you may stop your program once you reach your goal. *The purpose of exercise is to improve the quality of your life. You work out for the way it makes you feel: The internal results are primary, the external results are secondary.* A psychologist friend of mine routinely prescribes exercise for all of her patients, and she herself works out five times a week to "keep from going crazy."

Excuses, Excuses, Excuses

When it comes to reasons for not exercising, believe me, I've heard them all! For some, the word *exercise* conjures up visions of sweaty bodies, of people with tears in their eyes and pain plastered across their faces—and these torturous visions are used as excuses for not exercising. Exercise is about working your body to create positive results; it's not about self-destruction. If this is your vision of exercise, then you need to reprogram your mind to think of exercise in terms of movement, recreation, activity, and fun. Think of putting on your leotard or your gym shorts as one of the most positive *activities* in your day—one that will make you feel better, help relieve stress, and give you the energy and enthusiasm to function more effectively. *Exercise today for what it will do for you tomorrow.*

Then there are the "I can't afford to exercise" and "I don't have time to exercise" excuses. Guess what? *Economics and/or lack of time is no excuse for being out of shape.* First, don't tell me you can't *afford* to exercise, because I don't want to hear it. What does it cost to push the baby in her stroller for thirty minutes, run around with the kids at the park, take a walk, chop wood, mow the lawn, vacuum, hike, or ride a bike? These are all activities that translate into *exercise:* Your body doesn't know the difference. Get outside and move—get your blood flowing and your heart pumping! If it's a more structured exercise environment you're after, then investigate some of the community-service or fitness programs available in your area. *You don't have to belong to an expensive health facility to be fit.* Fat is fat—your metabolic system doesn't care how you burn it!

Second, *anyone* can find the time to exercise. I mean, if the president can fit it into his or her schedule, don't you think you can fit it into yours? *Make exercise a high-priority activity and plan for it ahead of time.* Get out your calendar and schedule an appointment with yourself to exercise. You wouldn't break an appointment with an important person, would you? Of course not! Aren't you worth it? You bet you are! To yourself, you are the most important person there is. The famous writer/poet Maya Angelou says, "Self-love, not selfish love, is the best feeling you can have about yourself." She's right.

Exercise Physiology 101

Before you begin designing an exercise program that's right for you, it's a good idea to learn some basics about exercise physiology: how your body responds to exercise, which type of exercise it needs, and what benefits you can expect to receive from exercising regularly.

In order for your body to change shape, you must make it perform certain activities. There are two types of training/exercise activities that your body responds to: aerobic and anaerobic. Each activity creates a different result, but they're all based on one principle: overload. Overload refers to specific training elements such as intensity, frequency, mode, and duration and can be muscle specific or refer to your body's overall metabolic responses to an activity.

Aerobic Exercise

Aerobic exercise requires oxygen to sustain it, whether it's a half an hour on a stationary bike or four hours in a road race. The best aerobic exercises are low to moderate in intensity and involve large muscle groups in continuous, systemic movement for a mimimum of 20 minutes. As your body performs an aerobic activity, the type of energy that it uses changes. During the first few minutes of continuous movement, most of your energy comes from carbohydrates (i.e., glycogen—stored body sugar). When your carbohydrate reserves become depleted, your body then begins calling up its fat reserves. Your body tells the fat reserves that it can't believe you're still *moving* so quickly and asks that some of the Crisco around your waist be released in the form of fatty acids, which it then breaks down into energy. Thus, the longer you perform an aerobic exercise, the more fat is needed and the more of it you'll burn. To sustain an aerobic activity without becoming fatigued, pace yourself: Go slower and go longer. Examples of good aerobic exercises are: walking, jogging or running, step aerobics or aerobic dance, swimming, stationary and open-road cycling, rowing, cross-country skiing, roller-blading, and rebound minitrampolines.

If fat burning is your goal, remember: You can't *melt* it off (it burns at 190 degrees) and you can't *rub* it off (remember all my loofah sponges?). *You've got to move it to lose it!*

Anaerobic Exercise

Anaerobic exercises, on the other hand, are those that do not require oxygen for movement. (Anaerobic means "without oxygen.") Anaerobic exercises tire you quickly and consist of short, quick bouts of movement; *however, they do not burn stored fat.* Because you're not moving for any consistent length of time, your body is able to perform anaerobic activities without drawing upon its fat reserves. The "stop and go movement" of anaerobic activities gives your body sufficient time to regroup and continue relying mainly on carbohydrates for its energy. That is why, for example, you can play straight sets of tennis every other day and still not lose any weight (body fat). Because tennis is an activity that does not require the continuous, nonstop movement of a strictly aerobic activity, your body seldom gets the opportunity to begin eating up its fat reserves. It can get by just fine on the carbohydrates.

Most recreational or team-sport activities fall somewhere in between aerobic and anaerobic, but lean more toward the anaerobic category. Some examples are downhill skiing, tennis, racquetball, baseball, and basketball. Yes, these exercises are strenuous and tiring, and they can burn calories and build endurance, but don't expect to burn a high percentage of fat and improve your body's overall composition through these exercises alone.

Again, if your primary goal is to burn fat, stay with the longer, less-intense aerobic exercises listed above. If you enjoy anaerobic recreational or team activities, don't give them up; just alternate them with aerobic, fat-burning activities. You can have your tennis games on

Tuesday and Thursday, but on Monday, Wednesday, and Friday jump on the stationary bike for thirty minutes instead.

Reaping the Benefits of Exercise

If you're still not convinced that you need to exercise, take a look at this list of hard-hitting facts regarding the benefits of regular exercise:

FACT: REGULAR EXERCISE WILL...

1. Eliminate unwanted (subcutaneous, visible) fat!
2. Strengthen bones and assist in prevention of osteoporosis (bone deterioration). Do you want to be walking around with your neck slumped forward and a hump in your back when you're sixty-five?
3. Increase your energy level. Higher levels of oxygen in your blood give you more energy throughout the day—no more complaining that you're "too tired" to work out!
4. Aid in transporting more oxygen to your brain, making thinking and decision making clearer.
5. Serve as a tool for battling depression and decreasing stress.
6. Improve your sleeping habits.
7. Improve your blood pressure and help fight heart disease.
8. Improve your circulation and digestion.

By now the message should be clear: *Get up and get moving!*

Crosstraining — Choosing What's Right for You

One year during high school I participated in track and dance. I remember that the assistant track coach pushed me to run faster and more aggressively by barking at me, "Stop running like a girl!" Then when I went to dance class, my instructor wrinkled her nose, shook her head, and called out to me, "Victoria! Be light, be graceful, stop jumping like a boy!" I felt like a tennis ball constantly bouncing back and forth between track and dance. Confused, frustrated, and unable to find a balance between the two, I finally gave up track and focused instead on my dancing. It wasn't until years later that I realized I actually *could* be a dancer and teach aerobics and at the same time push my body to its physical limits through sports such as running or bodybuilding. In fact, exercise research has proven that *variety is best*, and variety is the main principle behind *crosstraining*. Crosstraining— the concept of performing many different exercises or activities (versus strictly aerobic or anaerobic activities, for example)—accomplishes several things. First, it is the best defense against injuries due to overuse of muscles and joints. Second, it's also the best defense against boredom. Third, crosstraining is the most effective way to achieve a balanced exercise program—one that enhances your overall fitness level *and* your total physique.

If you're in the process of devising an exercise program, my advice is this: Choose from a variety of activities that you *like* (otherwise your motivation level is in trouble right from start) and choose from activities that build the following: strength, endurance, agility, coordination, and flexibility. Try to perform your activities at least every other day, and for a minimum of thirty minutes. After you become more comfortable with the activity and your fitness level improves, you can graduate to forty-five minutes to an hour and perform the activity four to five times a week.

Determining Intensity

Remember that popular sixties phrase "Bop 'til you drop!"? When it comes to exercise in the nineties, the message is definitely *Don't* bop 'til you drop! Take all things in moderation. How hard you work out depends on many factors, such as your age, your current health status and level of fitness, and your general fitness goals. Your heart is a muscle—a cardiac muscle—and it needs to be worked just as consistently as all the other muscles in your body. The most traditional method of monitoring and regulating exercise intensity is by checking your heart rate two or three times during your workout to determine how many times per minute your heart is beating. To check your pulse, *gently* place one or two fingers on your wrist or on one of the large (carotid) arteries on the side of your neck. Here are a few other guidelines that you should follow:

1. A ten-second heart rate is most widely used and considered the most accurate. Count the number of heart beats in a ten-second period and multiply that number by six to come up with your working heart rate (your exercising heart rate). Keep moving while you're counting—but make sure that you count your heartbeat, not your footsteps or the beats in the music.

2. The recommended (target) range for a working heart rate (fat-burning rate) is 120 to 160 beats per minute. The older you are, the lower your fat-burning range. Here's a heart-rate chart that you can use as your guide.

OPTIMUM TRAINING HEART RATES
DURING EXERCISE

▲ AGE	▲ MAXIMUM HEART RATE	▲ GENERAL POPULATION 65–80% OF MAXIMUM TRAINING RANGE	▲ FIT ATHLETE 85% OF MAXIMUM TRAINING RATE
20	200	130–160	170
25	195	127–156	166

▲ AGE	▲ MAXIMUM HEART RATE	▲ GENERAL POPULATION 65–80% OF MAXIMUM TRAINING RANGE	▲ FIT ATHLETE 85% OF MAXIMUM TRAINING RATE
35	185	120–148	157
40	180	117–144	153
45	175	114–140	149
50	170	111–136	145
55	165	107–132	140
60	160	104–128	136
65+	150	98–120	128

Karvonen Formula for Estimating Heart Rate:

220 - Age - Resting Heart Rate x Intensity + Resting Heart Rate = Training Rate

This method is considered the best for calculating your true working heart rate.

Heart-rate Formula: calculated at 70% training range.

220 - your age = theoretical maximum heart rate (TMHR).

Let's pretend I'm 40. My resting heart rate (RHR) is 50.

220 - 40 = 180 (TMHR).

Next you take your TMHR, subtract RHR to equal your Heart Rate Reserve (HRR).

180 - 50 = 130

70% of 130 = 91

To the 91 add 50 (RHR) for 141 OTR (Optimum Training Rate).

If you are on certain medications such as beta blockers, your heart rate numbers can be deceiving and not entirely accurate. For this reason, I prefer to use another method of monitoring exercise intensity: Perceived Exertion or Rate of Perceived Exertion (RPE). RPE involves a rating system based on a scale of zero to ten and translates how hard you *feel* (perceive) you are exercising. RPE makes *you*, not a fixed chart, responsible for monitoring workout intensity. Zero equals no movement—standing completely still—and ten is the equivalent of sprinting or being out of breath. A recommended range on the RPE scale is five to seven. A six on the RPE scale means that you're working at a challenging level, but you're not out of breath. (If you're out of breath, you won't be able to sustain the activity for very long.) At level six your breathing is steady and you're able to carry on a conversation.

Remember that thirty continuous minutes is the minimum amount of time you should spend exercising. However, the results of your workout will vary depending upon two factors. First, the length of the workout and, second, the intensity of the workout. If you're new to exercise and have a lot of fat you want to burn, you should work out longer (up to one hour) and at a lower intensity (lower RPE level). This will burn more fat, build up your strength, and reduce the risk of injury. As you gain strength and experience, you can reduce the time spent exercising if you increase the intensity of your workouts. It's time to move ahead when your workout becomes too easy. If you don't feel it, you're not getting the benefits you should. Increase the duration or difficulty—push yourself!

CATEGORY-RATIO RPE SCALE

0	Nothing at all	5	Strong
0.5	Very, very weak	6	
1	Very weak	7	Very strong
2	Weak	8	
3	Moderate	9	
4	Somewhat strong	10	Very, very strong; maximal

Whether you choose to monitor your workouts via a heart-rate chart or the RPE method, every twelve weeks you should take your pulse to determine your resting heart rate. *Your resting heart rate is ulti-*

mately *what determines the effectiveness of your exercise program*. The best time to check your resting heart rate is when you wake up in the morning (*after* you've recovered from the initial shock of your alarm ringing and your heart has stopped pounding). Locate your pulse on either your wrist or your neck, then count the beats for *one full minute*. The number that you come up with is your resting-heart-rate goal—it's how many times your heart should be beating at the end of your workout, after you've cooled down properly. If you're making progress with your exercise program, over time your resting heart rate should be lower. The lower your heart rate, the more efficiently you heart is functioning and the healthier you are.

Finally, in case you're wondering if there's a "best time to exercise," I don't really think there is. *Any* time is the best time to exercise—as long as you do it! Some experts would disagree with me, but I believe the key is really to find a time that works best for you. I mean, if you can't make exercise compatible with your life-style, you're not going to do it, right? Don't set unrealistic goals for yourself, and don't become discouraged if you don't see immediate results. Stick with your program and you will. Have your body fat tested regularly and track your resting heart rate. Both are great indicators of the overall success of your training program.

Remember: You didn't get *out* of shape in one week, so don't expect to get *in* shape in one week, either, okay?

▼

The chains of habit are generally too small to be felt until they are too strong to be broken. Make exercise a habit.

THREE SAMPLE CROSSTRAINING PROGRAMS:

1) Monday, Wednesday, Friday: Walk for 30 minutes. Tuesday, Thursday, Saturday: Body sculpting for 30 minutes.
2) Monday, Wednesday, Friday: New Step Workout with floor work for 30 minutes.
   Tuesday: Tennis.

Saturday: Technifunk™ Dance Workout with abdominal floor work for 40 minutes.

3) Monday: Walk the dog for 30 minutes.

Tuesday: Vacuum vigorously for 30 minutes.

Wednesday: Mow the lawn for 50 minutes.

Thursday: Stationary bike for 30 minutes.

Saturday: Hike or take a walking tour.

In the space below, start developing your own crosstraining program. As you learn about my three signature workouts later on in the book, make a goal for yourself to incorporate at least one of them into your new program. Whatever activities you choose, the message is move, move, move! Move with energy, excitement, and enthusiasm. Move with *attitude!*

MY CROSSTRAINING PROGRAM

DAY	ACTIVITY	DURATION
Monday		
Tuesday		
Wednesday		
Thursday		
Friday		
Saturday		
Sunday		

Chapter Six:
First Get Hot, Then Chill Out

Before you begin any type of aerobic conditioning workout, you must prepare your body by warming up and stretching. The main purpose of the warm-up is to prepare your muscles and joints for continuous, strenuous movement. Warming up increases your body's core temperature, which in turn increases blood flow to the working muscles and allows for more efficient energy production and utilization. Also, through the warm-up you increase the elasticity of your muscles— and the more elasticity your muscles have, the less likely you are to get injured during your workout.

My warm-ups are composed of slow rhythmic movements and specific muscle-isolation stretches (preparation stretches). These stretches are designed to give muscles more elasticity and flexibility, and each one should be held for six to ten seconds (eight to sixteen counts of music). The entire warm-up and stretch should last approximately eight to ten minutes. If you're a beginner, you may wish to warm up longer, and even if you're an intermediate or advanced exerciser, I still recommend that you perform the complete warm-up. Once you've warmed up and stretched properly, you can proceed with your aerobic activity.

After your aerobic activity, it's time to chill out and cool down your body. It's important that you keep moving during a cool-down so that your body returns *gradually* to its natural state. Continued movement also helps prevent the pooling of blood. Concentration of blood in one part of the body can cause stress to your metabolic system— you may feel dizzy, faint, or nauseated.

I use the same rhythmic movements for the cool-down as I do in the warm-up, then proceed to flexibility stretches. *Never go to the floor to perform stretches or floor work until your breathing is calm and steady.* If you're using a heart rate as your guide, don't lie down on the floor until your heart rate is 100 or less.

Flexibility stretches are held longer than preparation stretches and should not be performed during the warm-up because your muscles aren't warm enough to hold them for the recommended fifteen to thirty seconds per position. Each stretch series should be done four times per stretch. *Don't confuse the warm-up preparation stretches (six to ten seconds) with the flexibility stretches (fifteen to forty seconds).*

Using music in the warm-up and cool-down will make them more rhythmic and help your body move and flow more gently and naturally. Remember to select quiet, soothing music for your cool-down floor work and flex stretches. Here are some guidelines:

1. Be gentle—flow from stretch to stretch smoothly. Avoid sudden, jerky movements.
2. Stretch only to the point of tension in the muscles and joints, not to the point of pain.

3. Everyone has different levels of fitness and flexibility. Know what yours are and work within your limitations. *Never force a stretch.* If you become sore from stretching, back off and rest for a couple of days. When you resume your stretching, work up to more advanced stretches gradually.

4. Don't allow a partner to help you increase your flexibility by pushing you unless you are both trained in proper stretching techniques.

5. Never hold your breath. Use breathing to enhance your stretching. Exhale as you perform the lengthening movements.

6. *Most important, don't skip the warm-up, cool-down, or stretches even if you're short on time. Just reduce the number of sets in each series.*

Keeping an Attitude

During your warm-up and cool-down is the perfect time to call up some of the Life Training Tips from Part One.

As you warm up and prepare for your workout, take long cleansing breaths of oxygen. Inhale for two seconds, feeling your chest rise, and exhale for four seconds through your nose and mouth. The oxygen will give you renewed energy and clear the cobwebs in your head. With each breath you take, your body becomes stronger. *Visualize* enjoying your workout and the positive effects you're about to experience. Feel your blood begin to circulate at a rapid rate. See it race through your body carrying all the life-sustaining nutrients to your cells. Your sensitivity to movement translates into a heightened state of body awareness—focus your internal energy on the results that you're going to achieve by movement. *Establish a mind/body connection from the beginning of your workout and carry it all the way through to the end.*

When you perform your preparation stretches, maintain control of your movements—exhale through the lengthening phase and make them controlled and smooth. Repeat simple words to yourself to create positive emotions within, to motivate and excite you about what you're about to achieve. As you inhale, say the following: "Positive energy in. I have so much energy right now—I can't wait to start moving and sweating! Today I will walk faster, feel more powerful and in control. I love my life, and I'm excited to be alive. . . ."

In the cool-down, relax and slowly come down from the excitement and tension of your workout. Change your focus to more peaceful, calming thoughts. Now is when proper breathing technique is crucial. Inhale for two seconds, hold your breath for two seconds, then exhale for four seconds. As you breathe in and out, you are cleansing your entire system. Feel your blood moving more slowly along its path through your body, traveling to and from each limb and clearing away waste products created by your system during your workout.

Your muscles are now warm and supple—they're ready for your flexibility stretches. As you stretch, repeat to yourself: "That was a terrific workout—I'm proud of myself! What I just accomplished no one can take away from me. I close my eyes and reflect on the positive feelings of my workout. I see myself smiling, laughing, sweating, moving with power and conviction. I have just taken another positive step toward health and toward my life's training. Now as I go on with my day, I am more centered and balanced. I speak more softly and treat others and myself more gently and with more respect. I believe in myself and my ability to accomplish whatever I set out to do in life. . . ."

Let the Music Move You

In all the following three workouts there is one element that can make them either fun and exciting or tedious and boring. That element is *music*. Something mystical and magical happens when you listen to music. Music stimulates a wide range of feelings and emotions: It can make you happy, sad, calm, tense, sensual, or even enraged. Before you try these workouts, be selective about the music you choose. Look for positive, upbeat songs—songs that motivate you and make you want to move and groove during your sweat session. When it's time to cool down, switch to soothing, relaxing songs. *Make sure the music enhances, not detracts, from your workout.*

The Warm-up

Preparation for Workout

NOTE:
When looking at the photos throughout the workout sections, be sure to follow the corresponding captions word for word. My image will be a mirror image of you. That is, when I tell you to move your right foot, I will actually be moving my left foot; when I tell you to lift your left arm, I will actually be lifting my right arm. Use the photos to help check for proper form and body alignment, but use the captions for specific directions on how to perform each movement. Don't forget to breathe rhythmically throughout the entire workout. Never hold your breath. Keep your abdominals tight, your lower back controlled, and your upper body lifted.

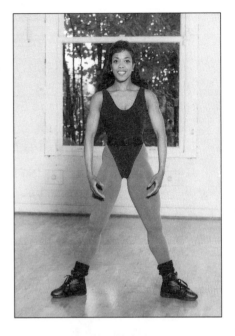

PREPARATION

1. Second position. Stand with feet beyond shoulder width, heels rotated forward, toes out at angle, pelvis tilted forward, shoulders back. Chest and torso are lifted. Do not sink into hip joints. Keep your weight centered over your pelvis.

DEEP BREATHING

1. With arms crossing chest, plié and inhale.

2. Extend arms overhead, shoulders down, back lifted, and straighten legs. Exhale and arms return to starting position. Repeat 4 times.

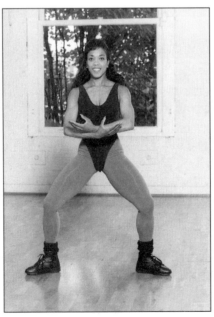

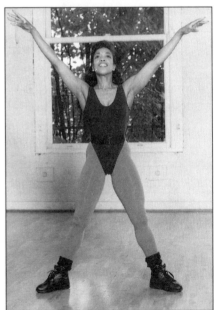

Rhythmic Warm-up and Jazz Isolations

Pelvic Tilt

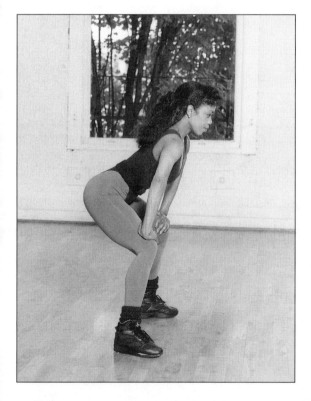 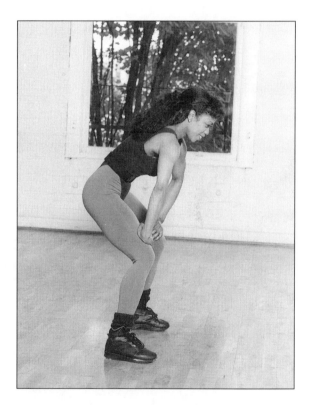

1. Place hands gently on thighs (above knees), isolate pelvis, and contract abdominals.

2. Tilt pelvis, contract abdominals and chest, separate upper back muscles, stretch lower back muscles. Hold for 4 counts and release. Do not stick your butt out. Repeat 8 times.

Pelvic Tilt with Spine Isolation

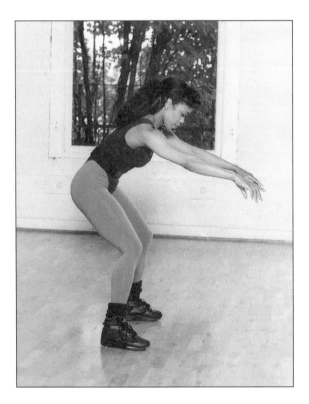

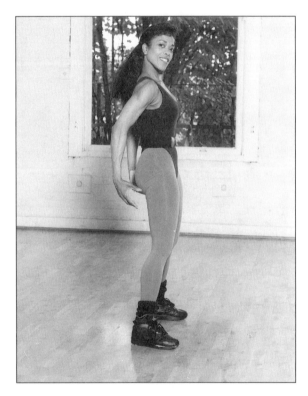

1. Arms extend front, abdominals tight, tilt pelvis—2 counts.

2. Chest expands, back contracts, arms release behind spine—2 counts. Repeat 8 times.

Shoulder Rotation

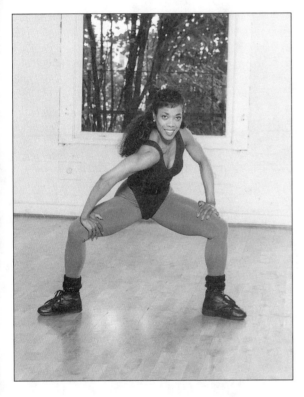

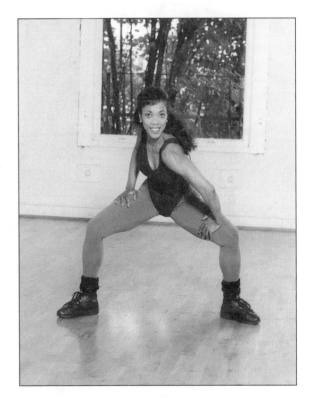

1. Second position plié, abdominals contracted, left shoulder rotates across torso, hands on thighs. Hold for 4 counts.

2. Repeat to opposite side. Hold for 4 counts. Repeat 4 times.

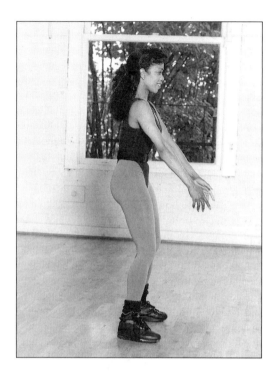

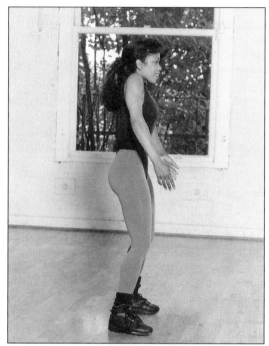

Shoulder Rolls

1. With arms to side, feet in wide second-position stance, gently roll shoulders back, breathe rhythmically—4 sets of 8 counts.

2. Repeat with shoulders rolling forward.

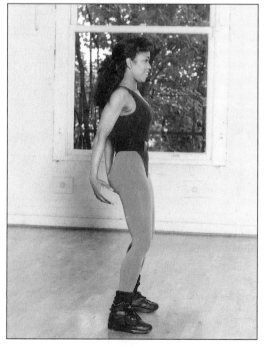

Torso Isolations

1. Feet parallel, right hand on abdominal wall, extend left arm, rib cage lifted. Shift from side to side, alternating arms. Repeat sequence 16 times.

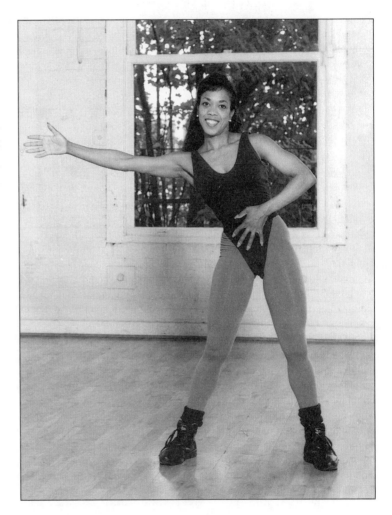

Rib Cage

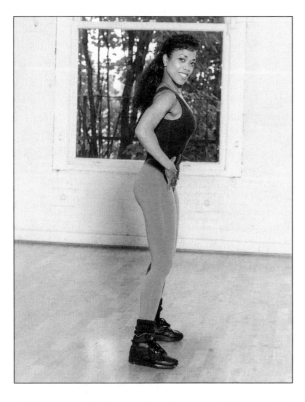 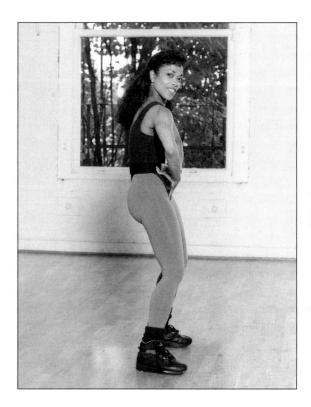

1. Feet parallel, jazz hands over abdominals, elbows to side, chest and rib cage expand forward.

2. Expand chest front, contract abdominals back. Don't sink into hips. Repeat for 16 counts.

Hip Isolation

Torso Stretch

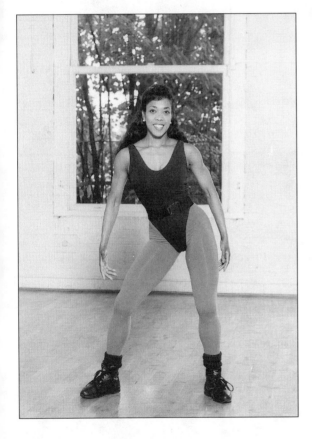

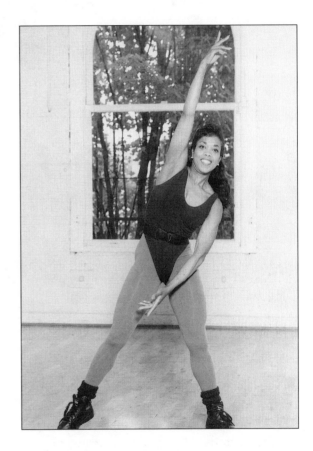

1. With arms to side, weight balanced over center of pelvis, rock hips from side to side. Control lower back, don't arch. Repeat for 16 counts.

1. Extend left arm over head stretching through waist, right arm crosses at waist, left toe points. Torso lifted off hips, keeping shoulders down, neck neutral. Repeat to right. Repeat for 16 counts.

Chest Cross

1. With one hand on waist, slightly turn hips and extend arm across body, abdominals contracted, soften knees, no torque on knee joints.

2. Repeat to opposite side. Repeat for 16 counts.

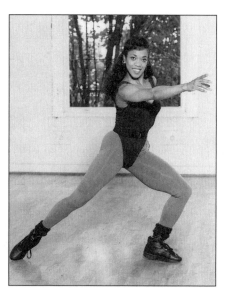
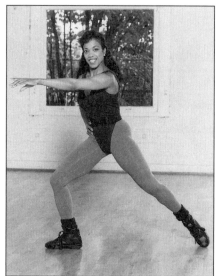

Parallel Passé

1. Feet parallel, pelvis tilted, arms extended forward, upper body contracted.

2. Knee flexed to rear, parallel passé, point toe, stay tall. Repeat sequence 8 times each leg.

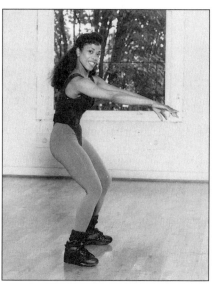
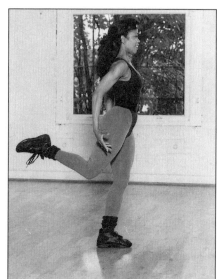

128

Bicep Curl/Hip Isolation

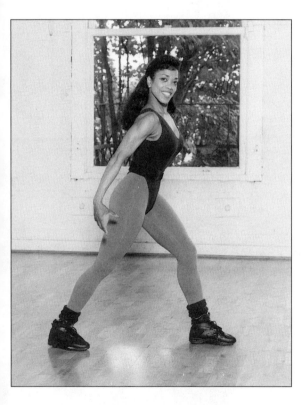 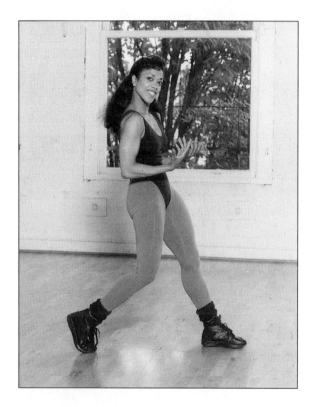

1. Stand in side lunge postion, hips and shoulders facing same direction. Arms back, abdominal wall tight.

2. Bring arms up in a bicep curl, gently flexing knee rolling through foot with heel lifting in back.

Isolation Static Stretch (Hamstring Stretch)

1. Right knee pliés, torso over hips, extend left leg front, left foot flexed, bend at torso. Hold for 8 counts. Repeat opposite side—2 sets per leg.

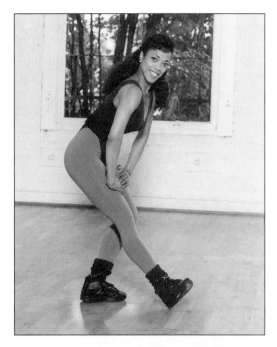

Calf Stretch

1. Legs staggered, both heels flat, upper body leaning forward—hold for 8 counts. Repeat on opposite leg—2 sets per leg.

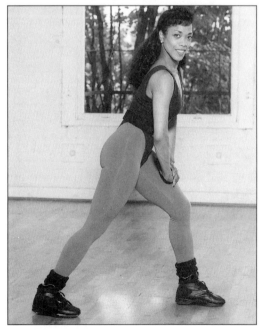

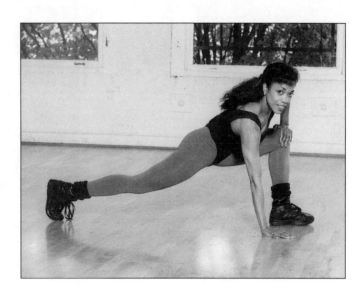

Runner's Lunge
(Quadricep Stretch)

1. In lunge position, right knee bent, right foot on diagonal (knee over heel), left leg extended. Left hand on floor, right hand on leg for support. Hold for 8 counts.

2. Left knee lowers to floor, torso upright, hands on thighs for support. Lengthen and stretch through left quadricep. Hold for 8 counts. Repeat #1 and #2—4 times each side.

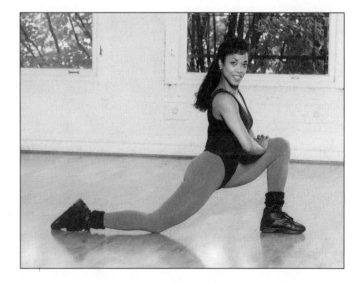

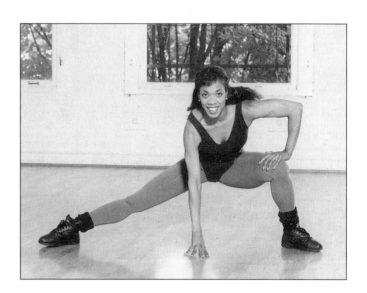

Groin Isolation Stretch (Advanced)

1. Facing forward, extend one leg to side, bend opposite leg at knee (aligned over heel), head stays above heart, hips pressed down. Transfer weight to opposite side. Hold for 8 counts. Repeat each side 4 times.

Anterior Shoulder Stretch

1. Feet parallel, clasp hands behind body and lift, opening up chest. Tilt pelvis forward slightly. Hold 8 counts, release. Repeat 2 times.

Posterior Shoulder Stretch

1. Repeat with hands clasped in front of body (opposite of anterior shoulder stretch). Hold 8 counts, release. Repeat 2 times.

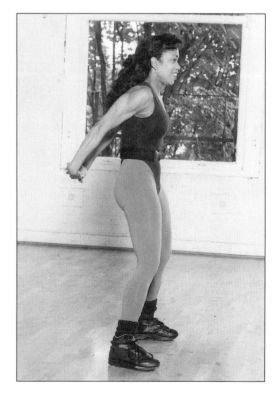

Head Tilt

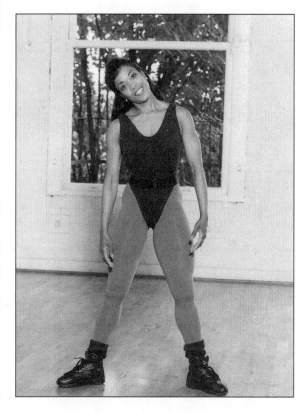

1. Gently lower head to one side, ear to shoulder. Maintain pelvic tilt. Hold 4 counts. Repeat both sides 4 times.

Chin to Chest

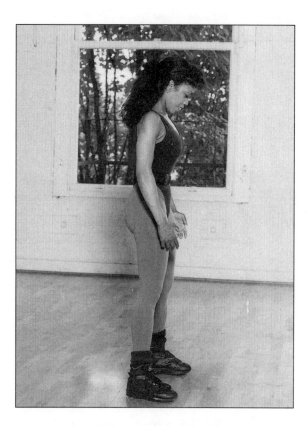

1. Gently lower head with chin down toward chest. Don't drop head rapidly. Hold 4 counts. Repeat 4 times.

The Cool-down Floor Isolations

Post cool-down: Once you have lowered your heart rate, you can move on to the body sculpting section of this book or perform Floor Isolations. **Refer back to warm-up stretches before going to Floor.**

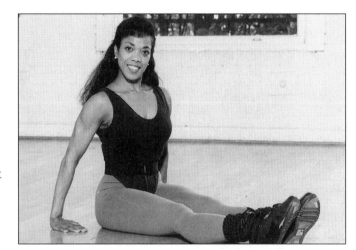

PREPARATION
1. Sit with toes pointed, shoulders back and down.

Inverted Hurdler Stretch

1. One leg extends with toe pointed, the other bends at knee with foot near the inside of knee of extended leg. Hands on floor in front or side of body. Lower chest toward extended leg and hold for 8 counts.

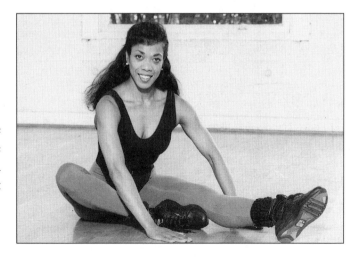

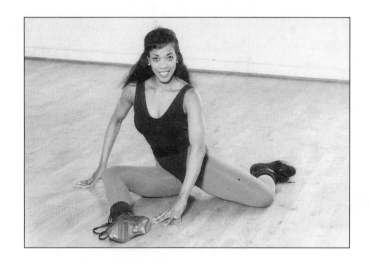

Front and Rear Attitude Stretch

1. Open front leg with knee slightly bent. Rear leg is bent loosely behind body. Hands positioned on floor near pelvis, hips squared off, abdominals contracted.

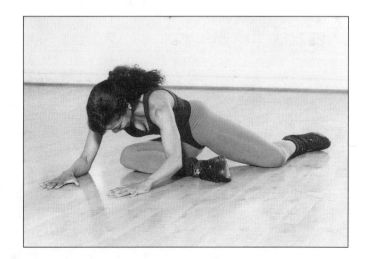

2. Lift up and over pelvis, legs relaxed and hands in front of body, lower torso toward the floor and hold for 8 counts.

Second Position Dancer's Stretch

1. Second position with toes pointed, pelvis tilted, hips squared, and hands supporting body behind hips.

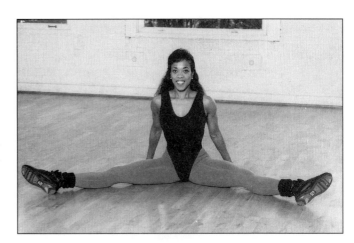

2. Rotate torso for a gentle stretch—repeat opposite side.

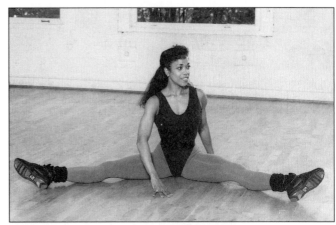

3. Lift one arm over head, reaching across body with opposite arm.

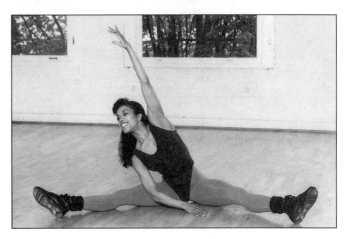

Crossover

1. On back, one knee bent, toes pointed, spine neutral.

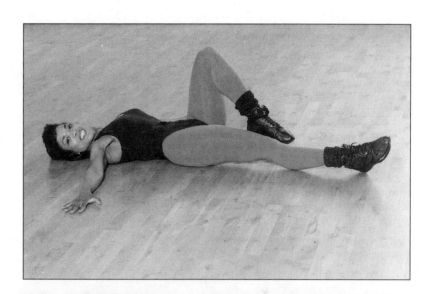

2. Bent knee crosses over, torso rotates, abdominals tight. Both shoulders remain on floor.

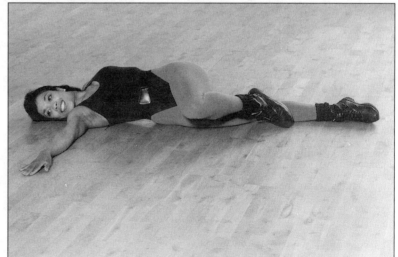

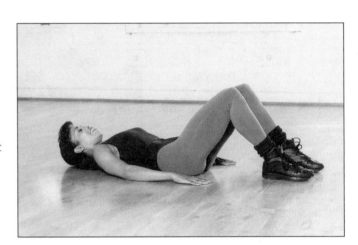

Hamstring Stretch on Floor

1. Lying on back, bend knees with feet flat on floor, pelvis neutral, arms at sides.

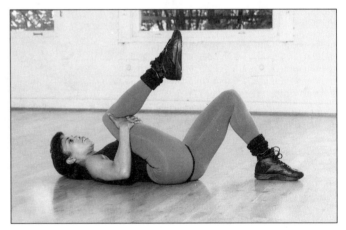

2. With one foot remaining on floor, bring one knee to chest, supporting leg at hamstring, abdominals tight, small of back pressed to floor. Hold stretch for 8 counts.

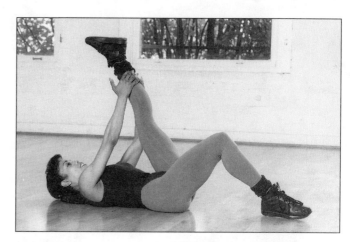

3. Extend leg and hold stretch for 8 counts. Repeat #1 and #2 with opposite leg.

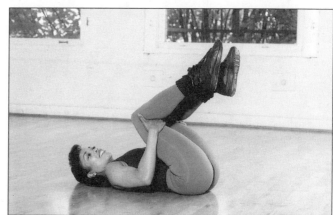

4. Bring both knees to chest, supporting legs at hamstrings, abdominals tight, small of back pressed to floor. Hold stretch for 8 counts.

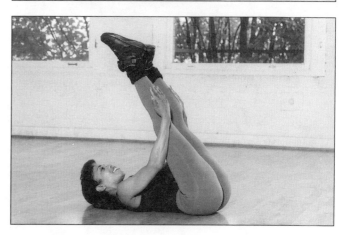

5. Extend both legs to ceiling, abdominals tight, small of back pressed to floor. Hold stretch for 8 counts.

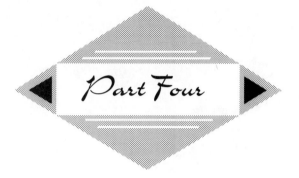

Part Four

THE NEW STEP
WORKOUT

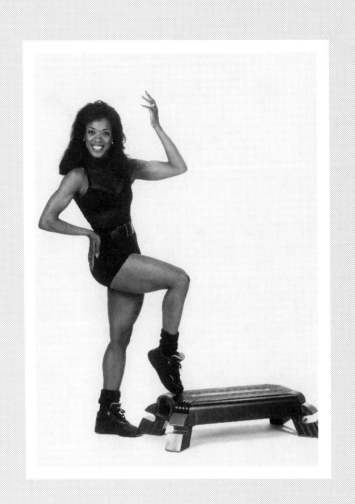

Chapter Seven:
Let's Get Steppin'

What Is Step Aerobics?

A spaceship lands outside an aerobic dance room on a Friday night. Through the windows, aliens watch in amazement as rows of sweaty earthlings step up and down and up and over simple platforms without *going* anywhere at all! The earthlings are grooving, clapping, and singing along to sounds never heard on Jupiter. What do you think the aliens would tell their buddies back home? "Not to worry, guys—there doesn't seem to be any real threat from Earth. Just a bunch of dripping earthlings stepping up and down on boxes and shouting something about 'Hammer time!'" *Hmmm . . .*

Although step aerobics probably *would* seem a bit strange to a visitor from Jupiter, those of us familiar with it know it's one of the latest and best developments to hit aerobics rooms and dance floors across the country. Step aerobics evolved about four years ago as an alternative to high-impact aerobics—the idea being to create a new, high-intensity, low-impact workout. Using a step platform, students performed simple up, up, down, down movements and arm combinations all set to slower aerobic music (kept between 118 to 120 beats per minute). At first, most students were using *ten-to-twelve-inch platforms* because it was believed that the higher the step, the more intense the workout. Not only was that early concept simply too intense for beginners, it was also no guarantee that a significantly higher percentage of fat would be burned. Plus, the higher platforms were responsible for numerous injuries to ankles, knees, lower backs, and Achilles tendons—not to mention that they built up quadricep muscles to the point where women began looking like linebackers! (The last thing *I* need is bigger thighs!)

In my classes I quickly moved to lower steps (six to eight inches), used music in the 124-beats-per-minute range, and began developing more dance patterns in combination with the basic step moves. (If you're tall and can maintain a safe 90-degree angle to your knees, then you can try a ten-to-twelve-inch step.) I also brought back more aerobic dance floor work—that is, I integrated more on-the-floor movements with the actual step routines (for example, a "grapevine" pattern on the floor and three step touches on the step platform).

Because step aerobics is still considered a new form of exercise, research regarding its overall effects continues. *Without doubt, however, it is one of the most effective ways to shape and firm up the lower body: hips, buns, thighs, and calves.* My feeling is that it's better to stick with a combination of aerobic dance *and* step workouts rather than perform basic step workouts exclusively. In keeping with the crosstraining philosophy, I recommend no more than four consecutive step workouts a week.

Are you ready? Let's get steppin'!

What You'll Need

You will need some kind of step platform to do the New Step Workout. (You can get a great workout using your stairs at home, too, and I'll tell you which moves you can use on your stairs later in this chapter.) There are many kinds of steps on the market today, and they range dramatically in price. Some are adjustable, others are not.

If you're new to step aerobics, an adjustable step may be best because it allows you to start low and increase the height as you become more advanced. Steps are available at most sporting-goods stores or large retail outlets.

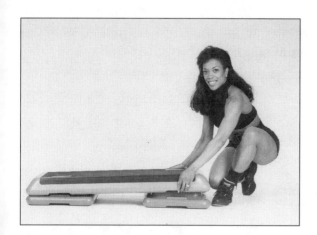

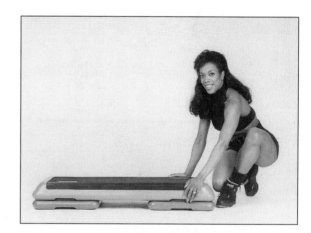

How High?

The height of your step corresponds directly with your fitness level, your height, and your step experience.

Beginner: Use a four-inch step (don't add any blocks). Stay with this height for at least eight to twelve weeks.

Intermediate and/or comfortable with step technique: Use a six-inch step. (This is the height I use.)

Advanced and/or very experienced with step technique: Use an eight-inch step.

Advanced and over 6 feet tall: Use a ten-to-twelve-inch step.

Which Tunes?

Step aerobics should be done to music that is high energy and has a strong beat. Funk music is very popular in step classes right now. Tune in a radio station that broadcasts top-forty songs, put on a favorite CD, or purchase specially mixed music available at record stores or through fitness organizations. For the New Step Workout, as well as for all of the workouts in this book, it will be important to determine how many beats per minute are in each of the songs you choose. Determining beats per minute is easy: simply put on your selections and count the beats for a total of one minute.

Beginner: Keep your music to 120 beats per minute.

Intermediate to Advanced: Keep your music to 122–126 beats per minute. *The maximum beats per minute for step aerobics is 126.*

My music philosophy for step is this: The higher the step, the slower the music.

Keep It Safe!

1. Consult your physician before beginning this or any exercise program.
2. Exercise with proper footwear, such as aerobic or crosstraining shoes. Don't wear running shoes: They have too much tread for the step.
3. Cotton clothing seems to work the best. It not only absorbs sweat well, but it also breathes and helps pull sweat away from your body. Don't wear heavy sweat suits—the workout is so intense that you could easily become overheated.
4. Warm up before your step workout and be sure to stretch your calves, quadriceps, hamstrings, and lower

back (see "Anatomy 101" in Chapter Ten).

5. When stepping up, be sure to place your foot on the middle of the step and emphasize pressing through the heel. Your heel should not hang off the step. Also, *step gently*—don't slam your foot down on the step.

6. Don't approach or mount the step while your back is facing the step.

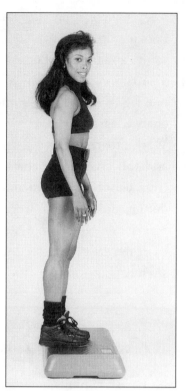
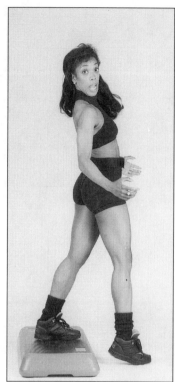

7. When stepping down, stay at a comfortable distance from the step (but not so far that you're leaning forward) and land with the ball of your foot and roll back onto your heel.

8. Keep your knees relaxed when stepping—don't lock them. Your knees should maintain at a 90-degree angle.

9. Don't step over the bench.

10. Maintain proper hip and knee alignment. Keep shoulders back, chest high, and pelvis tucked under.

11. Avoid pivoting movements on the step when the knee is loaded with body weight.

12. Don't rebound forcefully off the floor. Avoid ballistic stepping.

13. Keep your eye position steady during your workout. Looking up and down continuously causes nausea, neck strain, and fatigue of upper back muscles.

14. The maximum amount of time that you should work one leg (the lead leg) is one minute. After one minute, change legs.

15. Work progressively—learn the elements of movement and only change one at a time.

16. Keep your body hydrated. Drink plenty of water before, during, and after your workout.

17. Never just get off your step and stop moving for more than ten to twenty seconds. Cool down gradually and stretch.

No Step? No Problem!

If you don't have a commercially manufactured step or platform, you can still perform the New Step Workout using stairs inside or even outside of your home. The only moves that you won't be able to perform are lateral movements and ones that go over the top of the step. In fact, using your stairs at home is a great way to try the New Step Workout before committing to the purchase of a commercial step. On the following pages, all the moves and patterns with little steps ( ) next to them can be performed on your set of stairs.

The same safety rules apply to this workout that apply to the New Step Workout on the previous pages. Before getting started, measure the height of the step that you plan to use to make sure it's not higher than eight inches.

Chapter Eight:
Movements and Patterns

"If you don't squeeze your buns . . . no one else will!"

If you are looking for a balanced workout and are short on time, this New Step Workout is for you. The movements emphasize shaping the lower body as well as burning fat. The choreography is diverse, providing you with a multitude of movements that can be combined in a hundred different ways to create endless hours of step routines. This workout section is the most complete source you will ever see written on step aerobics.

Cuing Tips: If you are working out with an instructor, be it in a studio or with a video, there are counts and verbal commands that the instructor gives. Those commands are called "cues." I have included "cuing tips" throughout the workouts to assist you with your interpretation of the movements, combinations, and sequences.

Basic Step

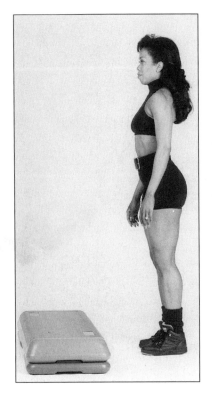 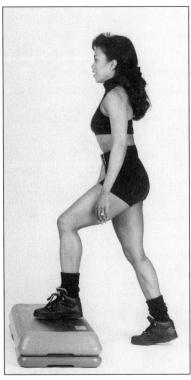 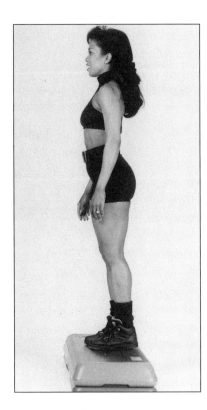

1. Stand with feet hip-width apart, facing step.

2. Step on platform with right foot.

3. Step on platform with left foot—both feet on top.

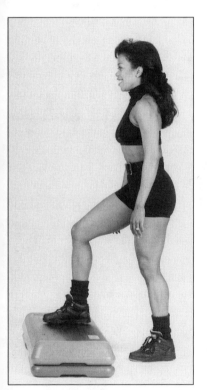

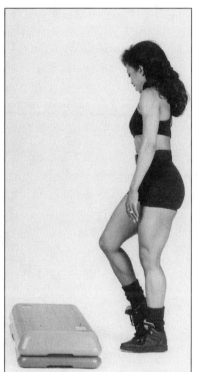

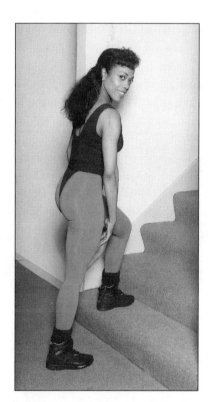

4. Step off platform with right foot.

5. Step off platform with left leg, back to starting position (arms swing naturally at your side as if walking).

Cuing tip: up, up, down, down.

Home Step Variation:
Same foot pattern as Basic Step.

Changing Feet

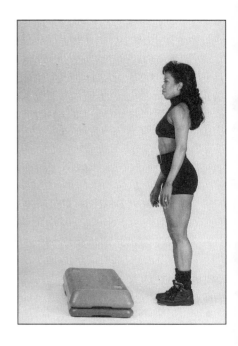

1. Stand with feet apart, facing platform.

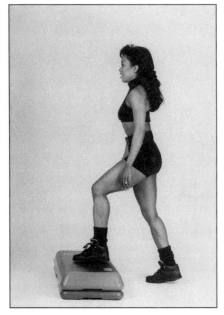

2. Step up on platform with right foot.

3. Step up on platform with left foot.

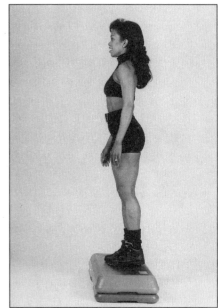

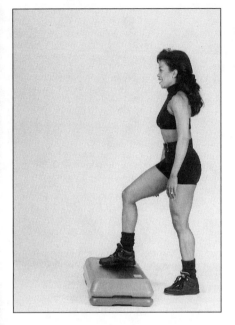
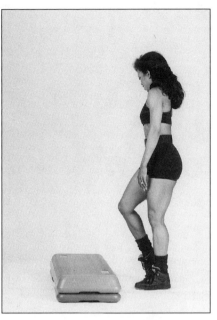

4. Step down off platform with right foot.

5. Left foot taps on floor.

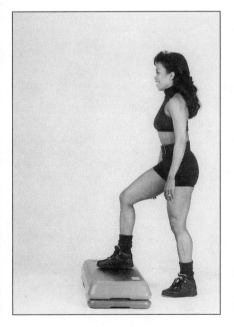
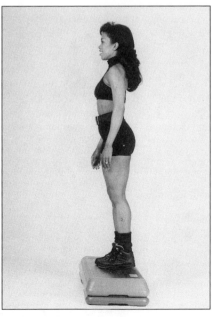

6. Step up on platform with left foot.

7. Step up on platform with right foot. Repeat this move stepping down off platform with left foot and tapping with right foot to change feet and work opposite leg. Switch back and forth as desired.

Cuing tip: up, up, down, tap and change.

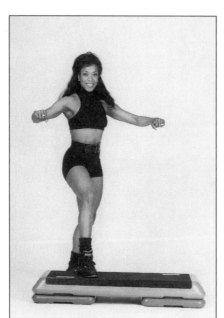
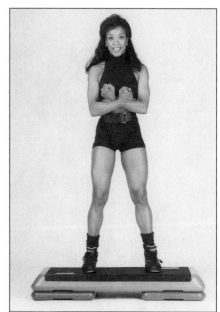

Walking Down (Inside Press)

1. Step up on platform with left foot, arms held out in lateral raised position.

2. Step up on platform with right foot, bring elbows together across chest.

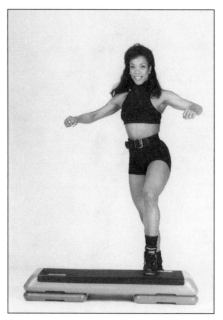
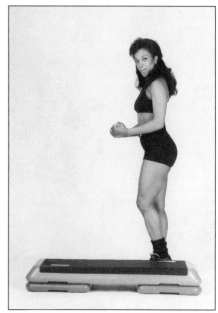

3. Step off platform with left foot, bring arms back.

4. Tap right foot back, push arms down.

154

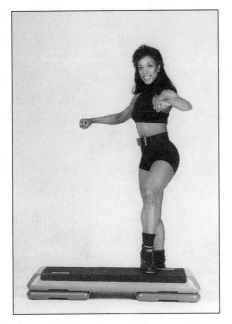

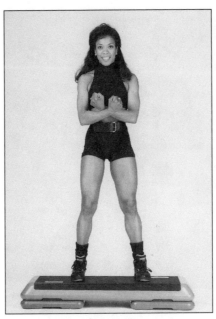

5. Step up on platform with right foot, arms go up in lateral raised position.

6. Step up on platform with left foot, press elbows across chest.

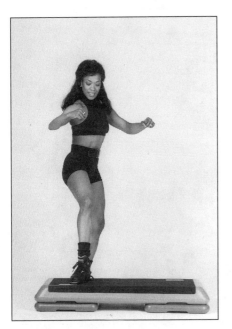

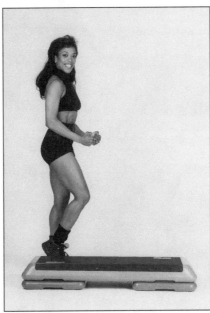

7. Step off platform with right foot, bring arms back.

8. Return left foot to floor, arms go down.

Repeat this move stepping down off platform with left foot and tapping with right foot to change feet and work opposite leg. Switch back and forth as desired.

Cuing tip: up, up, down, tap and change.

155

Walking Down with Wave

1. Step up on platform with left foot, arms bent at elbow as if you were carrying two trays.

2. Step up on platform with right foot, sweep arms in and cross chest.

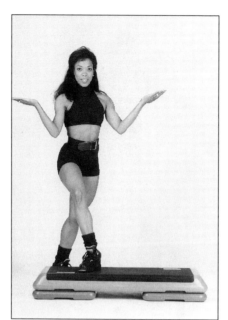
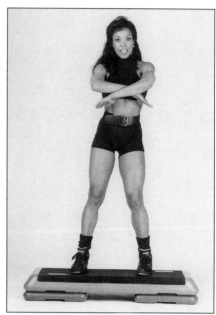

3. Step off platform with left foot, sweep arms back out to sides.

4. Tap right foot back, push arms down in front of body, crossing at wrists.

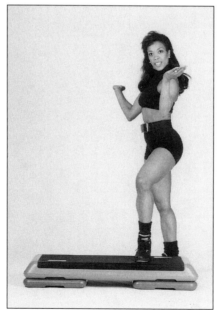
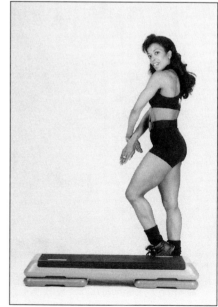

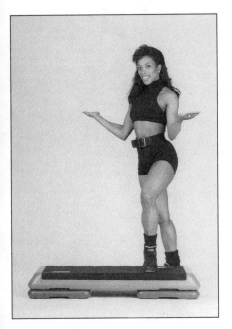

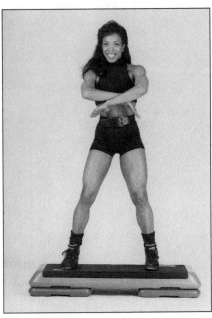

5. Step up on platform with right foot, arms bent at elbow as if you were carrying two trays.

6. Step up on platform with left foot, sweep arms in and cross chest.

7. Step off platform with right foot, sweep arms back out to sides keeping elbows tucked into sides.

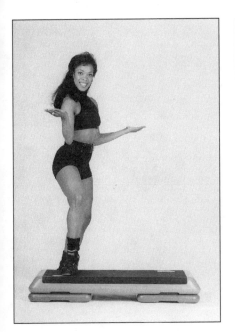

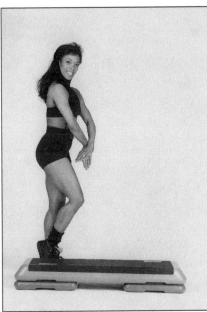

8. Return left foot to floor, push arms down in front of body, crossing at wrists.

Repeat this move stepping down off platform with left foot and tapping with right foot to change feet and work opposite leg. Switch back and forth as desired.

Cuing tip: left, right, left, tap right, right up. Arms: out, press, out, down.

157

Walking Down (Knee Lift or Ankle Touch) ▞

1. Step up on platform with left foot, arms held out in lateral raised position.

2. Step up on platform with right foot, bring elbows together across chest.

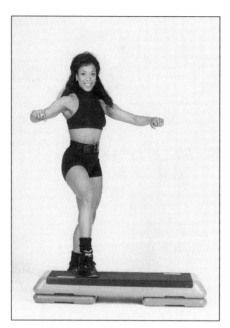 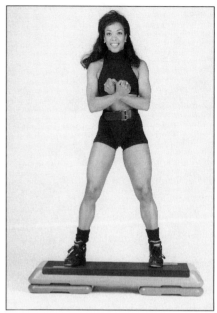

3. Step off platform with left foot, bring arms back.

4. Lift foot off platform, rotating left arm across chest to meet knee and curling bicep.

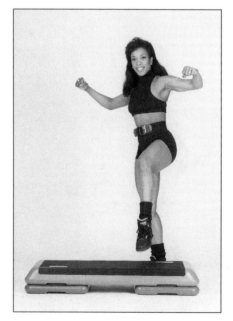 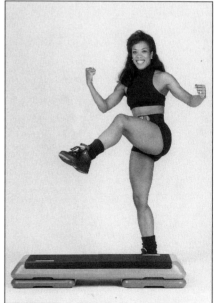

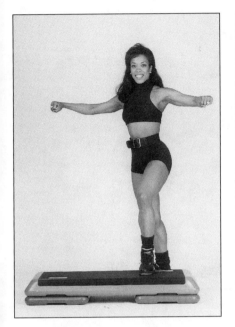
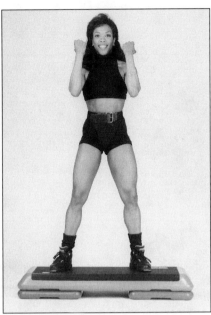

5. Step up on platform with right foot, arms go up in lateral raised position.

6. Step up on platform with left foot, press elbows in toward chest.

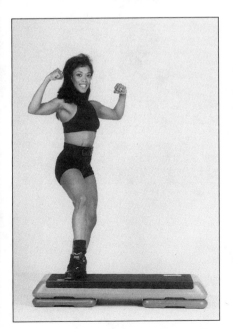
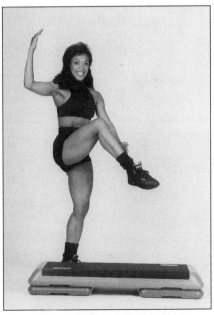

7. Step off platform with right foot, bring arms back.

8. Lift left knee, rotate torso to touch ankle with right hand, raise left arm out to side.

Repeat side to side.

Cuing tip: left, right, lift left. Arms: out, chest, out, touch ankle.

Step Touch
(Hold one side)

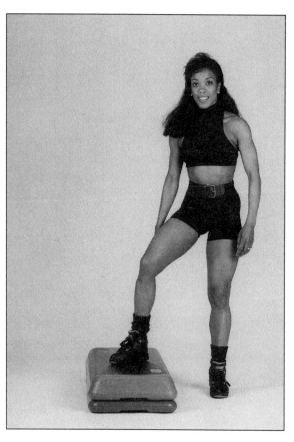 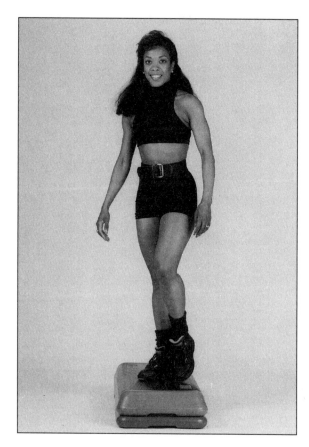

1. Step up on platform with left foot, with body at slight right angle.

2. Tap right foot on top of step

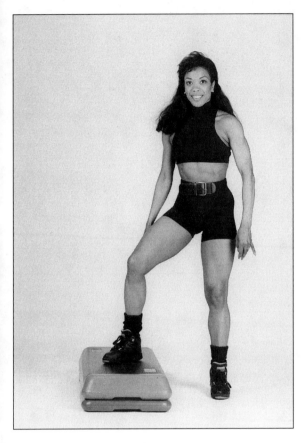

3. Step back to floor with right foot.

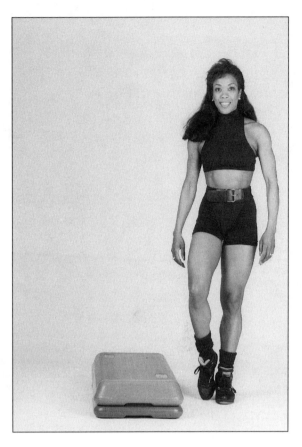

4. Bring left foot to floor.

Repeat to one side for approximately one minute and then switch to opposite side.

Cuing tip: step right, tap left, step left, tap right.

Step Touch Variations include: Arabesque, Hamstring Curl, Lateral Lift, and Window Wash.

Note: Maximum repetition one minute each leg.

161

Arabesque

1. Step up on platform with left foot, with body at slight right angle.

2. Lift right leg behind body—both arms lift.

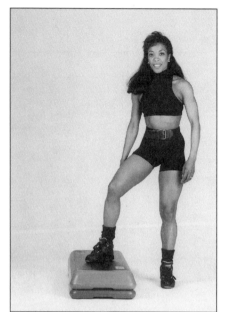
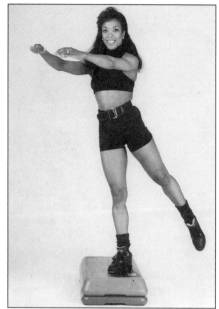

3. Step back to floor with right foot.

4. Bring left foot to floor.

Cuing tip: step Arabesque (or step lift), step touch.

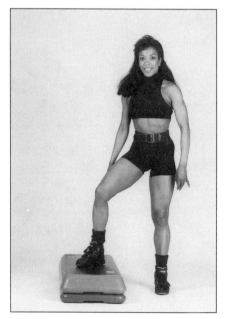
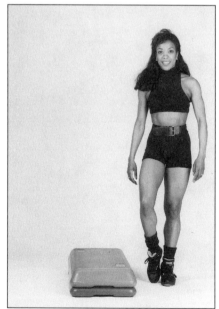

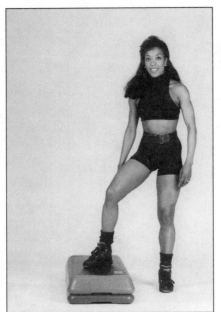

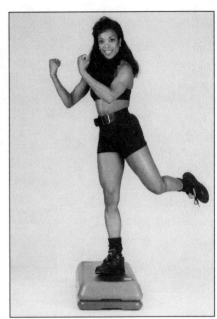

Hamstring Curl (Rear Attitude) ◢

1. Step up on platform with left foot, with body at slight right angle.

2. Bend right leg behind body in hamstring curl—arms lift in a bicep curl.

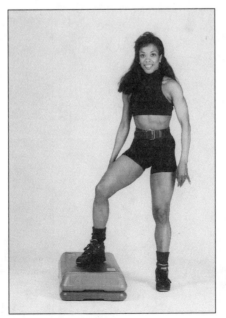

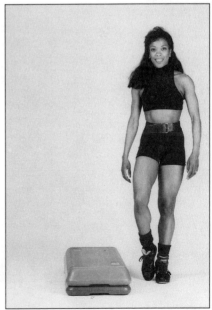

3. Step back to floor with right foot.

4. Bring left foot to floor.

Cuing tip: step curl, step touch.

Lateral Lift

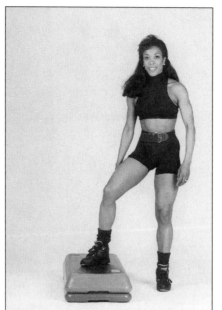
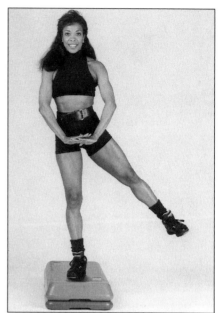

1. Step up on platform with left foot, with body at slight right angle.

2. Lift right leg to side in a lateral lift—arms push down in front.

3. Step back to floor with right foot.

4. Bring left foot to floor.

Cuing tip: step lift, step touch.

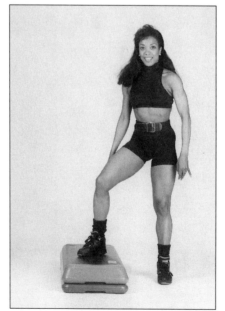
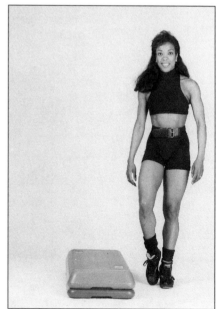

Window Wash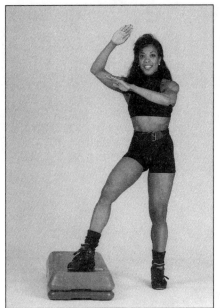

1–2. As you step up,
arms lift over the head
in circular pattern (as if
you were washing a
window).

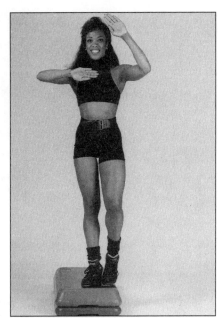

3–4. Stepping down,
press arms down by
sides.

Cuing tip: step and
wash, step and wash.

*Home Step Variation:
Same foot pattern as Step
Touch and Variations.*

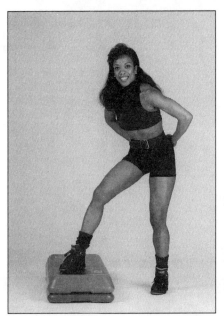

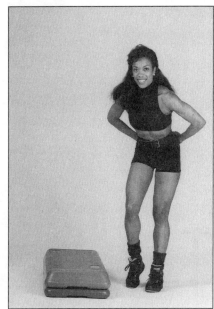

1. Demonstration of Arabesque.

2. Demonstration of Lateral Lift.

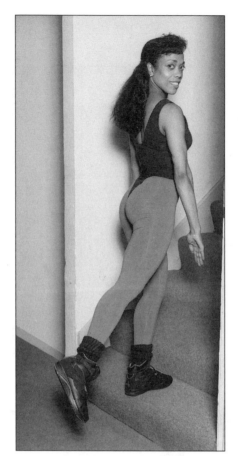 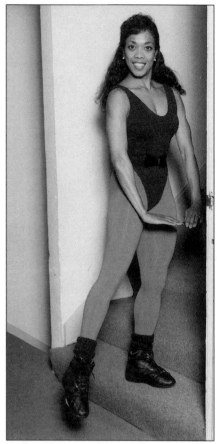

Over the Top — Dancer Arms

1. Stand parallel to step. Step up with left foot, torso rotates left, arms extend on diagonal.

2. Step up with right foot, arms close to front.

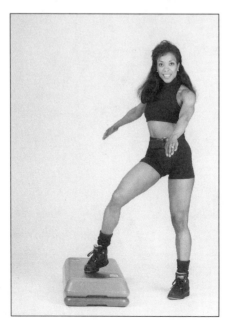 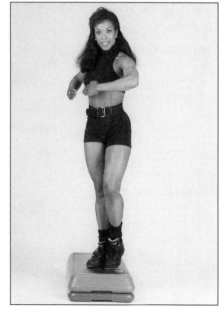

3. Step off with left foot (outside leg) on opposite side of step, upper body still rotated slightly on left diagonal, arms extend.

4. Step off with right foot (both feet now together), torso rotates to left and arms close back to center.

Repeat to other side, leading with right foot.

Cuing tip: step left, right, left, tap, up and over the top.

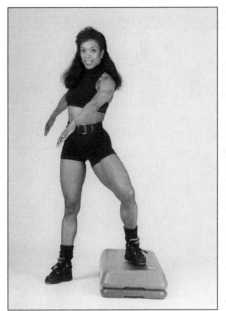
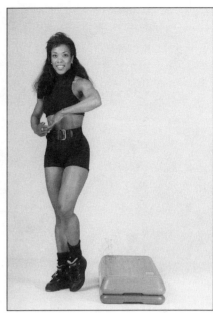

(These variations can be combined with walking your step to make a multitude of patterns and combinations.) *Variations to Over the Top include: Grapevine Behind and Turn Behind Step.*

Grapevine Behind

Repeat #1 through #4 of original Over the Top move.

5. Don't go back over step; instead, step wide behind step, arms extending laterally.

6. Cross right leg behind left, arms cross in front of body.

7. Step out with left foot, arms extending laterally.

8. Bring feet together. (You are now at the left side of step and can combine up and over with a walk behind step.)

(See photos of steps 5 through 8 on next page.)

Cuing tip: Over the Top, Grapevine Behind.

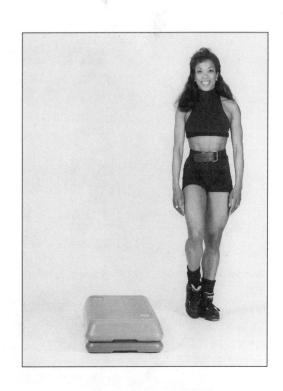

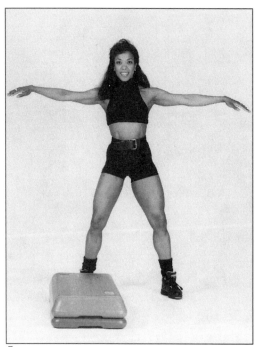

5

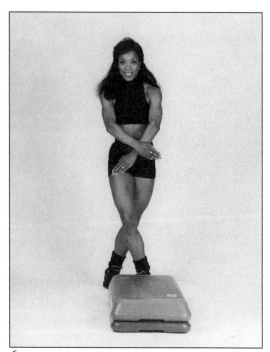

6

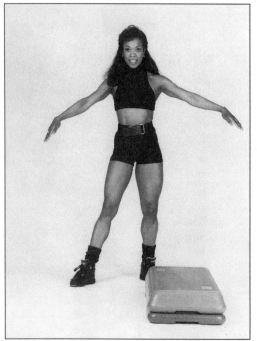

7

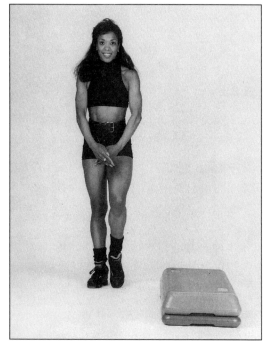

8

Chaîné Turn Behind Step

Repeat #1 through #4 of original Over the Top move.

5. Don't go back over step; instead, step wide on floor, jazz hands.

6. Half turn to left facing back with hands coming in over abdominals.

7. Half turn to face front again, arms back out to sides in jazz position.

8. Tap feet together, with hands coming in over abdominals. (You are now at the left side of step and can combine Over the Top with the Turn Behind Step.)

Cuing tip: Over the Top, Turn Behind.

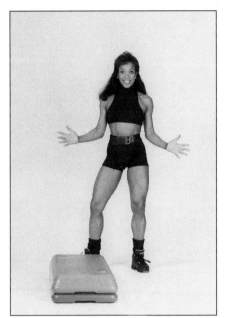
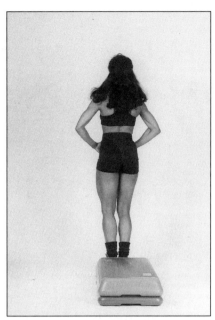
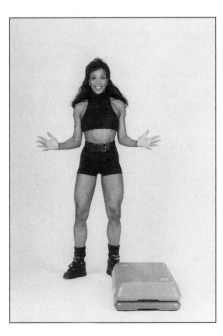
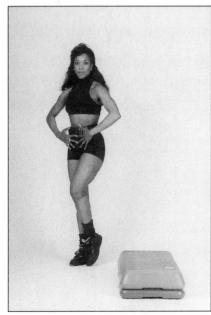

Step Straddles —Troop Arms

1. Both feet on top of platform with knees together.

2. Step off with left leg to begin straddle, shoulders lifted, arms bent at elbow and crossing body to left.

3. Step off with right leg to complete straddle, repeat arms to right.

4. Step back up with left leg, arms repeat left.

5. Step back with right leg, arms repeat right.

Repeat with right lead leg for approximately one minute, then alternate left.

Cuing tip: down, down, up, up. Arms: both arms — pump left, pump right, pump left, pump right.

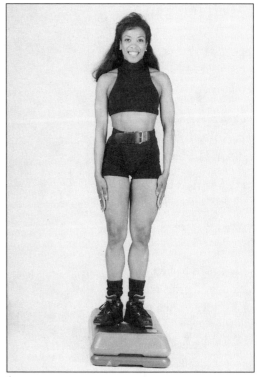

1

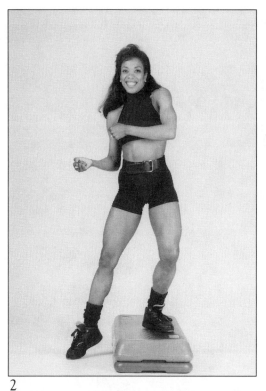

2

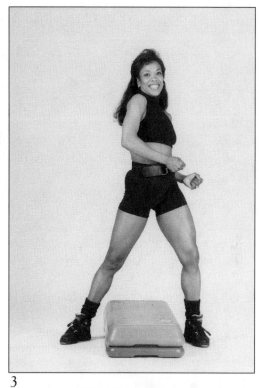

3

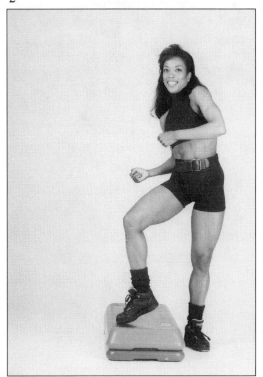

4

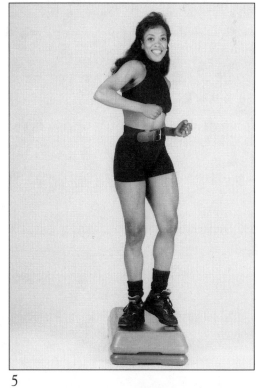

5

Alternating Step
Straddles — Vogue Arms

1. Starting position.

2. Straddle down left, left hand comes to right cheek.

3. Straddle down right, left hand comes to left cheek.

4. Step up with left leg, left arm extends, palm out.

5. Step up with right leg, left arm down at side, right hand remains on hip.

Repeat 2 to 4 on opposite side switching legs each time you return to top.

Cuing tip: down, down, up, tap. Arms: cheek, cheek, extend, down.

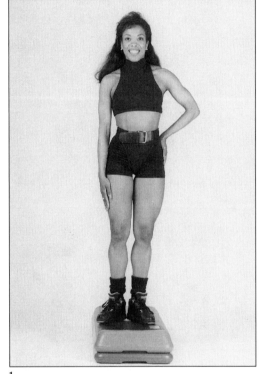

1

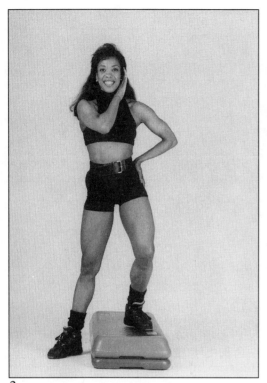

2

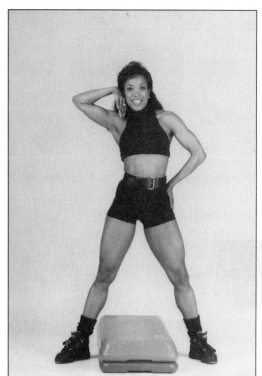

3

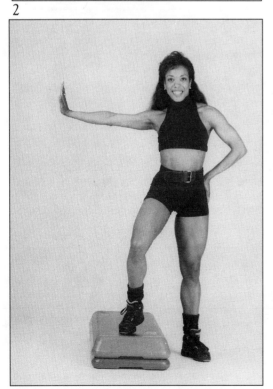

4

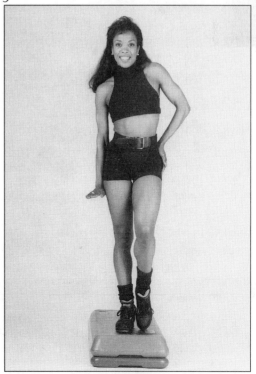

5

Funky Wave Over the Top

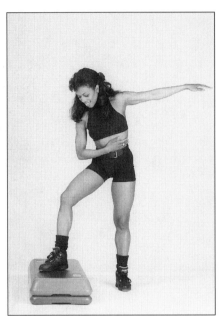
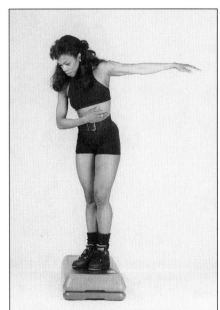

1. Beginning at right end, step up with left foot, left arm wrapped over abdominals, right arm waves behind.

2. Step up with right foot to meet left, arm continues to wave.

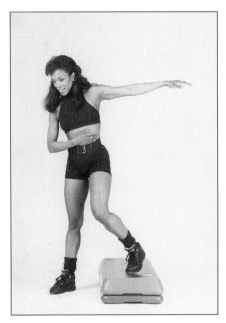
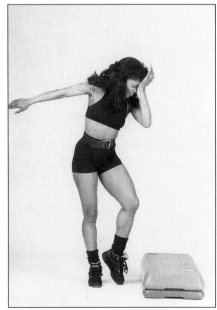

3. Left foot continues over and steps off left side.

4. Right foot taps on floor, left arm lifts behind body and right hand comes to head. Repeat other side.

Cuing tip: Over the Top. Arms: cross and wave.

Straddle Variations

In place of tap add following options:

1. Knee lift — cuing tip: step knee or front attitude.

2. Hamstring and bicep curl — cuing tip: step curl or step rear attitude.

3. Hip extension and arm lift — cuing tip: step lateral lift.

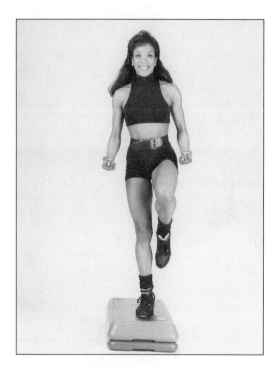

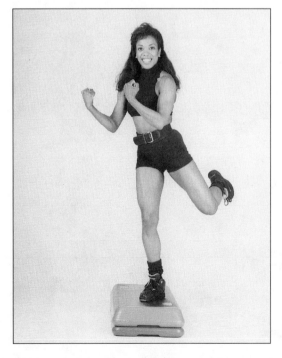

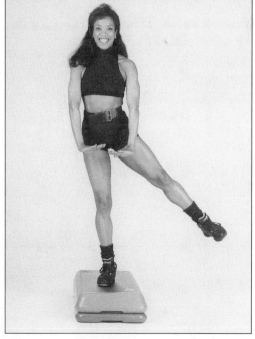

T-Step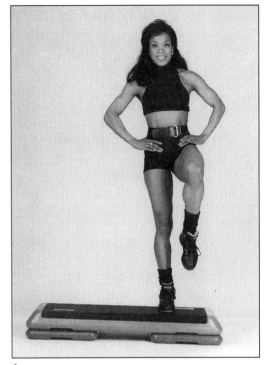

1. Left foot steps up, right knee lifts.

2. Right foot to floor, left foot taps step.

3. Repeat sequence #1 and #2.

4. Left foot steps wide on floor toward left side of step.

5. Right foot steps up, left knee lifts.

6. Left foot returns to floor, right foot taps step.

7. Repeat sequence #5 and #6.

8. Right foot steps wide toward right side of step.

Cuing tip: step knee, step knee, back, back, other end, step knee, step knee, back, back, other end.

T-Step Variations include: T-Step—Lateral and T-Step with Hip Rotation and Leg Extension.

1

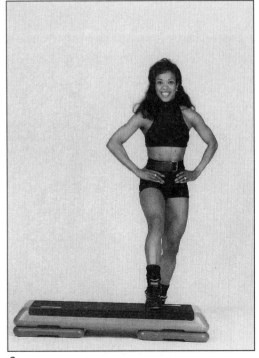

2

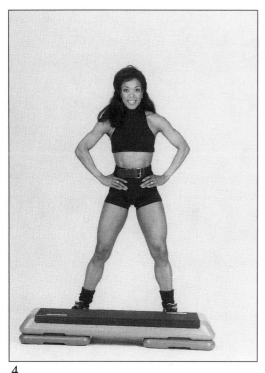

4

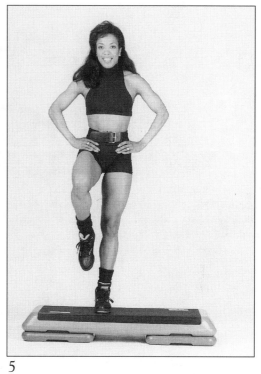

5

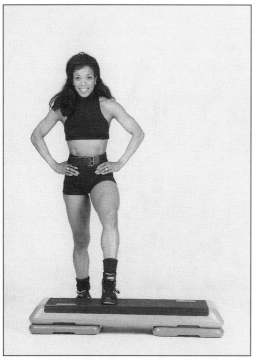

6

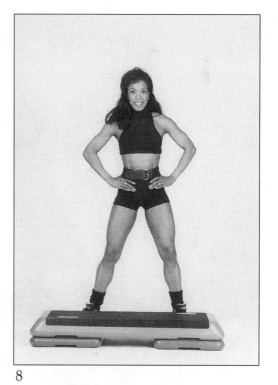

8

T-Step — Lateral

1. Right foot steps up.

2. Left knee lifts.

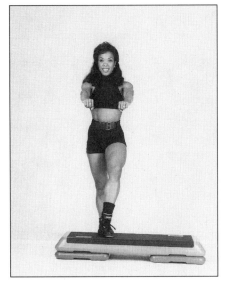
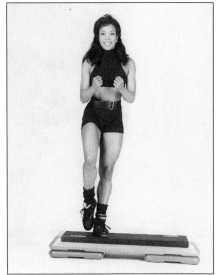

3. Left foot steps off left end of step.

4. Right foot steps off to meet left foot.

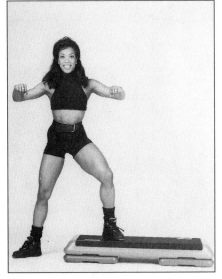
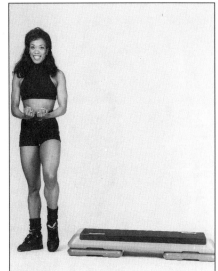

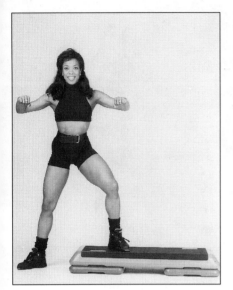

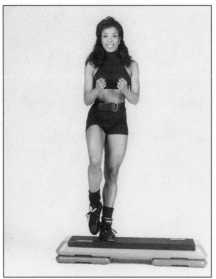

5. Right foot steps back up on end of step.

6. Left knee lifts.

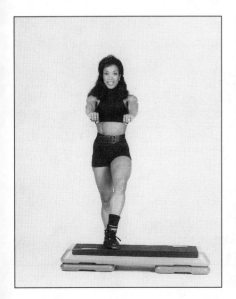

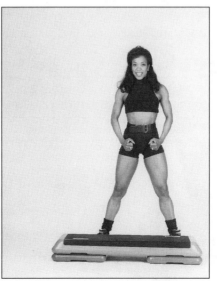

7. Left leg steps back.

8. Right foot steps wide to right end of step.

9. Left foot steps up.

10. Right knee lifts.

11. Right foot steps off right end of step.

Repeat motion to left.

Cuing tip: step lateral, step side, step knee, back, back, to other end.

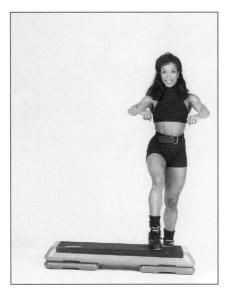
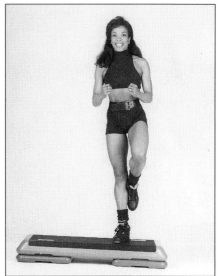
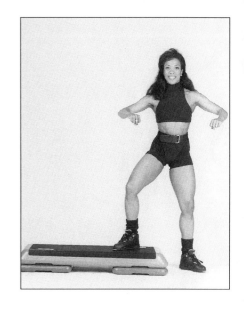

T-Step with Hip Rotation and Leg Extension (or Arabesque)

1. Right foot steps up.

2. Left knee lifts and hip and foot on step rotate in $1/4$ turn to right and arms lift overhead.

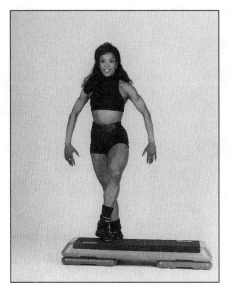
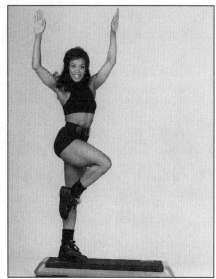

3. Left foot steps off left end of step, arms open side.

4. Right foot steps down to meet left foot.

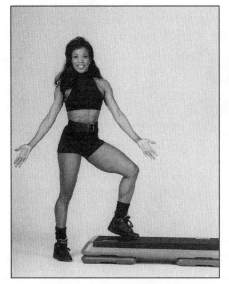
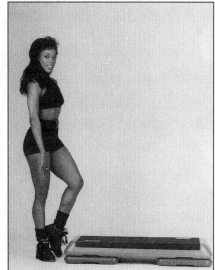

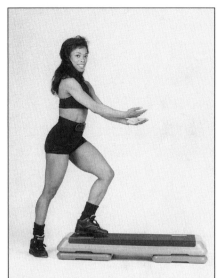 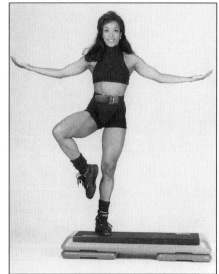

5. Right foot steps back up, arms sweep in front of body.

6. Left knee lifts and foot and hip rotate to passé, arms open.

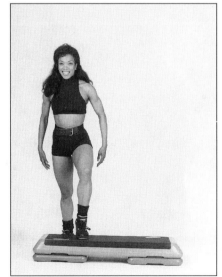 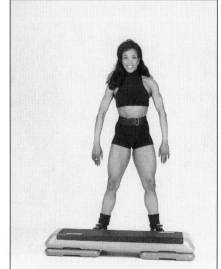

7. Left leg steps back, arms down to sides.

8. Right foot steps wide to right.

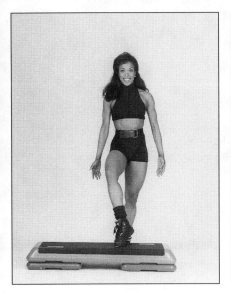

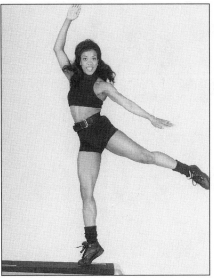

9. Left foot steps up.

10. Right leg extends and hip and foot rotate $1/4$ turns, arms in fourth position.

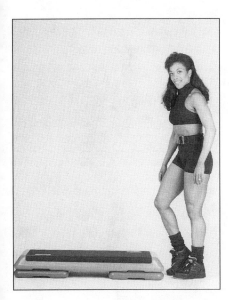

11. Right foot steps down off end of step and left foot taps.

Repeat motion to left.

Cuing tip: step $1/4$ turn, step touch, step $1/4$ turn, back, back.

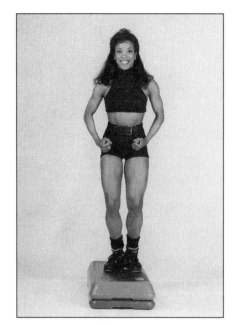
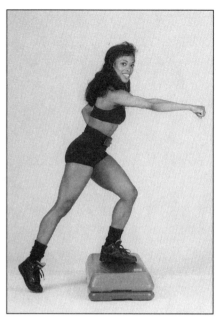

Power Shaping Moves

Lunges — (single and double)

1. Starting position with both feet on step.

2. On diagonal, lunge off step, left arm punches at diagonal.

3. Return both feet to step.

4. Alternate lunge, keeping left foot on step and lunge of side with right foot.

Cuing tip: tap down, right, left, right, left.

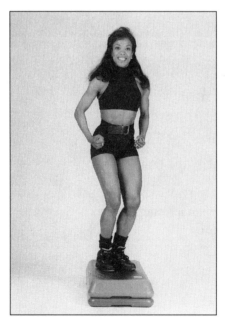
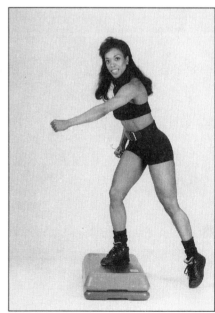

Power Leg Pumps

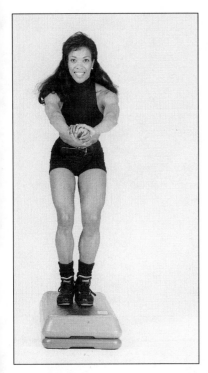 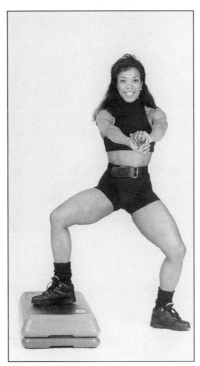 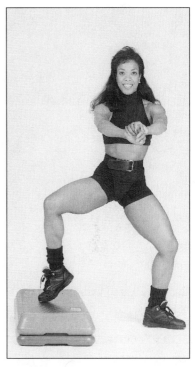

1. Both feet together on top of step, knees bent, feet flat, arms reaching to front.

2. Step right foot off to right of step beyond shoulder width apart, knees bent, back straight, shoulders lifted.

3. In plié, hands clasped, lift left heel and pulse down and up.

Repeat #1 to #3 to left side of step.

Cuing tip: center, right, press down, lift heel, press down.

Three Knees and Step Behind (no photos)

1. On right end of step, left foot steps up, right knee lifts, right foot steps back, left foot taps (repeat 3 times moving to left end of step).

Cuing tip: step, knee, step, tap; step, knee, step, tap; step, knee, step, tap; step, knee, step, tap.

2. Change directions, stepping up on left end 3 times moving to right end of step.

Three Knees and Step Behind Variations include: Slide Double Hop and Hammer.

Slide Double Hop

1. Left leg steps left, arms angle to sides.

2. Slide right to meet left leg, right arm sweeps with left leg.

3. With both feet together, hop up, arms at waist and pumping to left.

4. With both feet together, hop up again, arms at waist and pumping to right.

Cuing tip: step knee (3 times), slide on floor, hop.

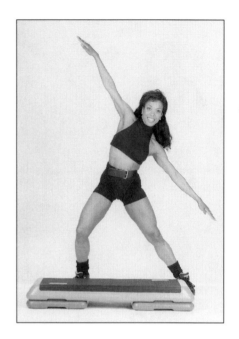

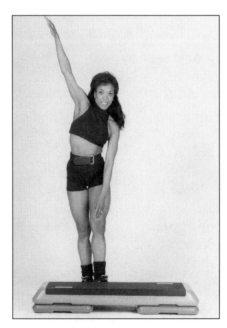

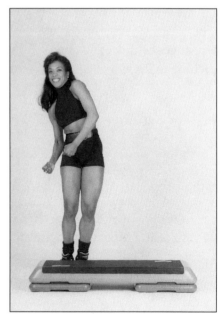

Hammer

1. At right end of step, left knee lifts and rotates to left, right arm is bent, hand is at shoulder in fist.

2. In one count, pump arm down to waist, left leg comes to floor, and right leg lifts behind.

3. Repeat #1 moving left.

4. Repeat #2. You will end your move at the left end of step.

Cuing tip: step knee (3 times), floor slide, lift, slide, lift.

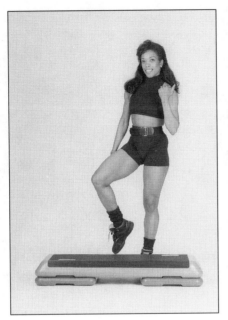
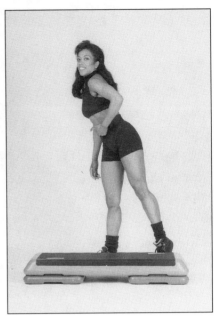
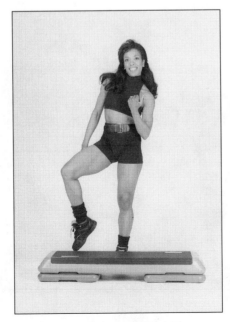
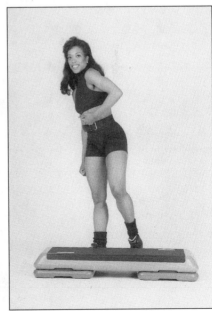

Pivot at End Step

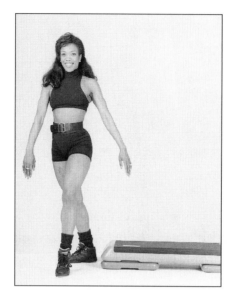
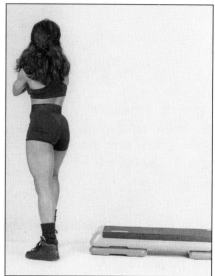

1. At left end of step, arms lift slightly to sides, right leg crosses left and steps forward.

2. In one count, pivot to back with feet remaining in position, hands come together across chest.

3. Facing the back wall, bring left foot across right, arms lift slightly to side.

4. In one count, pivot back to front with feet remaining in position.

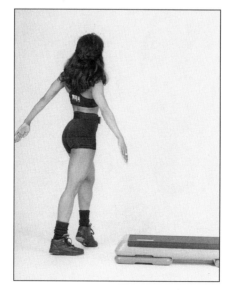
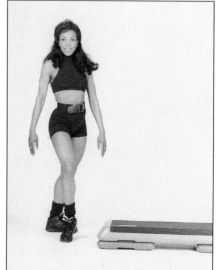

Hip-Hop Straddle

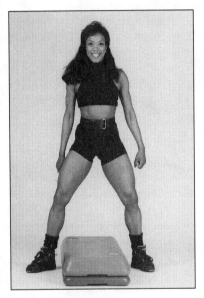 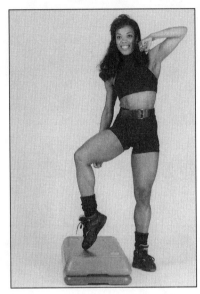 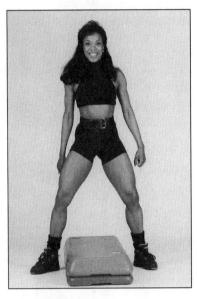

1. Both feet on floor straddling step at center.

2. Left foot taps step.

3. Left foot returns to floor.

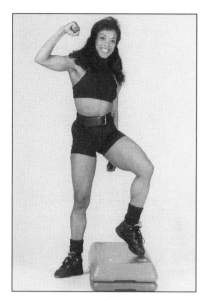

4. Right foot taps step.

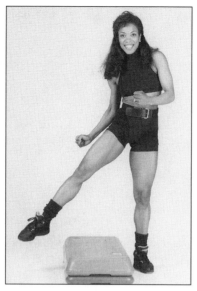

5. Right foot returns to floor and left foot lifts off floor and steps back down.

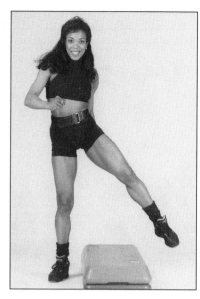

6. Right foot lifts off floor and steps back down.

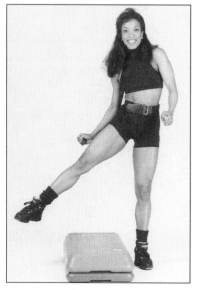

7. Repeat #5.

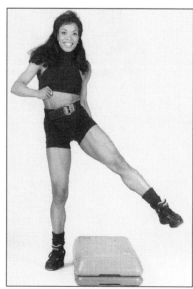

8. Repeat #6.

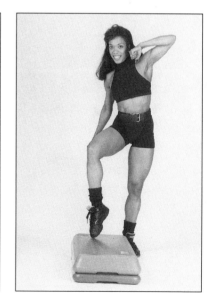

9. At end of step, left foot taps top of step and returns to floor.

Cuing tip: tap up, tap up, travel back.

Chug Forward

10. Coming forward, legs straddle step, right hand on abdominals, left arm out to side and bend at elbow, rib cage pressed forward.

11. In one count, pump arm down and contract ribs back, both feet scoot forward.

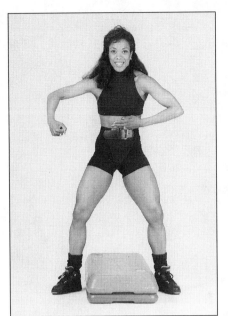
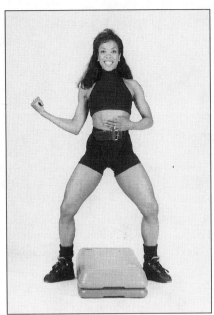

12. Repeat #10, with both feet scooting forward again.

13. Repeat #11 with both feet scooting forward for last time.

To continue this movement, simply begin at #1 and repeat the whole combination.

Cuing tip: hop 1, 2, 3, 4.

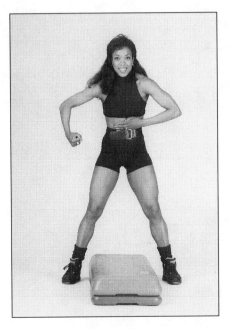
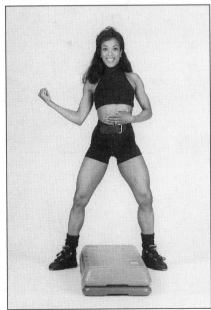

Body Sculpting on Step

Chest:

Basic Press

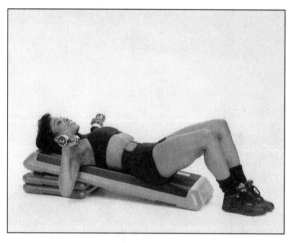

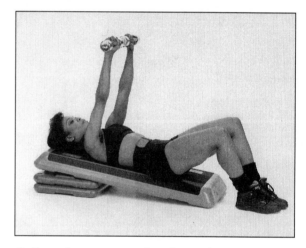

1. With step at incline, knees bent, feet flat on floor, elbows out to side, back flat on step.

2. Straighten arms, palms facing knees and contracting chest muscles (pectorals).

Chest Flys

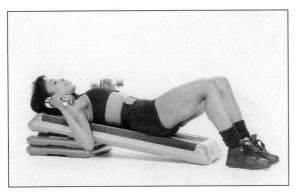

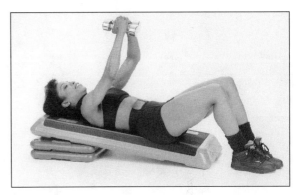

1. With step at incline, knees bent, feet flat on floor, elbows out to side, back flat on step, palms face center of body.

2. Bring palms together, maintaining slight bend through elbow and contracting chest muscles. Maintain elbow flexion throughout entire range of movement.

Pullover

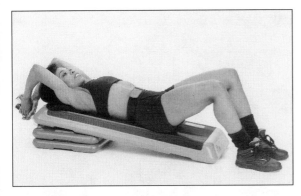

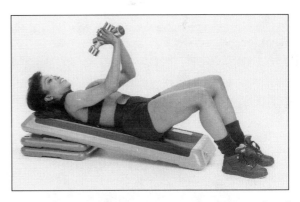

1. With step at incline, knees bent, feet flat on floor, elbows close to head and pointed to ceiling, palms close and facing each other. (Make sure you have a firm grip on your weights and head remains on step and back is flat on step.)

2. Maintain bent elbows, raise weight over head to center of chest, contracting abdominals and chest through entire range of movement.

Return to position and get a full stretch at end opening chest and lats.

Abdominals:

Basic Crunch

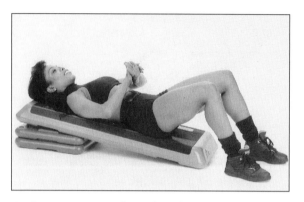

1. Step on an incline, hands clasped together over abdominals, knees bent, back flat, pelvis neutral.

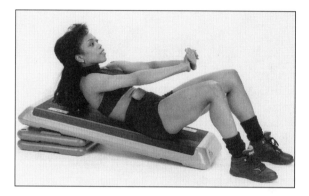

2. Roll shoulders off step and crunch. Hold 2 counts and return to starting position.

Crunches with Weights

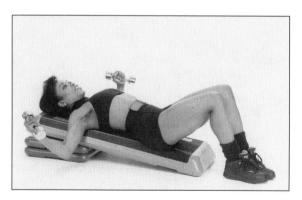

1. Step on an incline, elbows at side, palms at shoulders, knees bent, back flat, pelvis neutral.

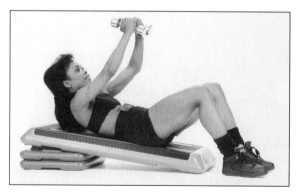

2. Abdominals crunch, bring hands together with shoulder blades raising off step.

Return to starting position.

Chapter Nine:
New Step Workouts

Level 1 — Beginner

Less is better if you are new to exercise. Too much at one time may discourage you or cause injuries. Fitness is a lifelong commitment.

If you are a beginner to exercise, start with a step that is four inches high and tailor your workout along the following time line:

Warm-up preparation and stretch: 8 to 10 minutes
Step workout: 10 to 15 minutes
Cool-down and flexibility stretch: 8 to 10 minutes

Level 2 — Intermediate

If you have been doing step aerobics for three months or are familiar with aerobic exercise (and you have no previous knee or back injuries) you are ready to use a step that is a little higher (six to eight inches).

Warm-up preparation and stretch: 8 to 10 minutes
Step workout: 20 to 40 minutes (do not exceed 40 minutes)
Cool-down and flexibility stretch: 10 minutes

At this point, you are gaining endurance, skill, and stamina. Be careful not to step continuously for more than forty minutes. Stepping longer than this can create overuse injuries.

Level 3 — Advanced

Now you are ready to challenge yourself with faster music (up to 126 beats per minute) and more complex choreography. Try using some of the arm patterns from the Body Sculpting chapter to create a more intense muscle-training workout with the step.

Be extremely careful about the height of your step. Many instructors push ten to twelve inches (if you are over six feet tall and fit, this may work for you). As I mentioned before, I usually use a four-to-six-inch step and get a great workout. A higher step does not necessarily mean a better workout, so find the height that is comfortable for your fitness level. Research being conducted on step aerobics throughout the country is showing that you get just as effective a workout without having to go to a higher step. Also, more students are confessing to injuries directly related to higher steps. It is better to remain on the conservative side than to compromise knees, joints, and body alignment.

Warm-up preparation and stretch: 8 to 10 minutes
Step workout: 20 to 40 minutes (don't exceed 40)
Cool-down and flexibility stretch: 10 minutes

Beginner — Intermediate — Advanced

The New Step Workout Outline

(Total Minutes: 35 to 50)

Warm-up preparation and stretch: 8 to 10 minutes
Repeat each movement 8 to 16 times.
(See Chapter Six for movement descriptions.)

Deep Breathing
Pelvic Tilt
Pelvic Tilt with Spine Isolation
Shoulder Rotation
Shoulder Rolls
Torso Isolations

JAZZ ISOLATION SERIES

Rib-Cage Isolation
Hip Isolation
Chest Cross
Parallel Passé
Bicep Curl/Hip Isolation

STATIC ISOLATION STRETCH

Runner's Lunge
Calf Stretch
Hamstring Isolation
Groin Isolation
Posterior Shoulder Stretch
Anterior Shoulder Stretch
Head Tilt
Chin to Chest

STEP WORKOUT: 10 TO 40 MINUTES

(See Chapter Six for movement descriptions.)
1. Basic Step: Right leg lead, repeat one minute.
2. Step Change
3. Basic Step: Left leg lead, repeat one minute.
4. Step Change:
Beginners: Repeat sequence one time.
Intermediate: Repeat sequences #1 through #4 three times.
Advanced: Repeat sequences #1 through #4 four times with arm variations from body-sculpting section.
5. Walking Down with Inside Press:
Beginners: Repeat 2 minutes. **Elapsed time: 6 minutes.**
Intermediate: Repeat 4 minutes adding variations: Walking Down with Wave, Knee Lift, or Ankle Touch. **Elapsed time: 12 minutes.**
Advanced: Repeat 4 minutes adding variations: Walking Down with Wave, Knee Lift, or Ankle Touch. **Elapsed time: 16 minutes.**

6. Step Touch:

Hold on one side 1 minute and repeat on opposite leg.

Beginners: Repeat 2 times adding variation of Hamstring Curl. **Elapsed time: 10 minutes.** (This is the end of beginner workout; continue with cool-down.)

Intermediate: Repeat each leg 4 times adding variations of Arabesque, Hamstring Curl, Lateral Lift, and Window Wash. **Elapsed time: 20 minutes.**

Advanced: Repeat each leg 4 times adding variations of Arabesque, Hamstring Curl, Lateral Lift, and Window Wash. **Elapsed time: 24 minutes.**

7. Over the Top — Dancer Arms:

Intermediate: Repeat each side 4 times, then add variations like Walking Behind, Turn Behind Step, Funky Wave Over. **Elapsed time: 25 minutes.**

Advanced: Repeat each side 4 times, then add variations including Walking Behind, Turn Behind Step, Funky Wave Over. **Elapsed time: 29 minutes.**

8. Bench Straddles:

Intermediate: Repeat each leg 1 minute each side adding variations including Troop Arms, Vogue Arms. **Elapsed time: 31 minutes.** (This is the end of Intermediate workout; continue with cool-down.)

Advanced: Repeat each leg 1 minute each side adding variations including Troop Arms, Vogue Arms. **Elapsed time: 34 minutes.**

9. Lunges (Alternating):

Advanced: Repeat lunge each side, 16 times.

Combine with straddle movement (#8). Repeat approximately 3 minutes. **Elapsed time: 37 minutes.**

10. Squats from Center of Step:

Advanced: Repeat 3 minutes.

Elapsed time: 40 minutes. (This is the end of advanced workout; continue with cool-down.)

COOL-DOWN:

Grapevine side to side — 1 minute
Chest Cross
Chest Press
Parallel Passé
Bicep Curl/Hip Isolation
Calf Stretch
Hamstring Isolation #1
Groin Isolation #2

This is the end of your step workout. Your options include moving on to specialty isolation stretches or going on to the Body Sculpting moves.

Final Note: This sample workout does not include all the moves outlined in the Step Moves section. As you become familiar with the workouts, simply add moves.

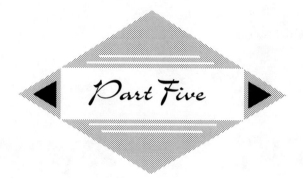

Part Five

THE BODY
SCULPTING
WORKOUT

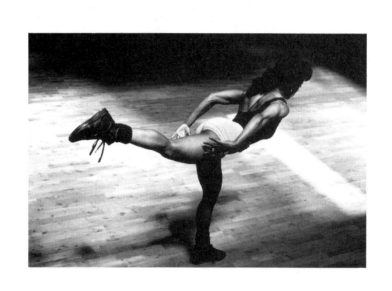

Chapter Ten:
Pump That Body

What Is Body Sculpting?

Gone are the days of Twiggy arms and Olive Oyl legs. Thank goodness being a "stick" is no longer fashionable. Today, one sign of a healthy, attractive woman is the strength of her muscles and the shape of her body. Women want their bodies to have shapes, curves, muscles, and *definition*. One of the most popular classes that I teach is my HABIT (Hips, Abs, Buns, and Incredible Thighs) class—a "definition workout" designed for both men and women. This is a low-impact workout designed to create strong, lean upper bodies and shapely, toned lower bodies through the use of light hand and leg weights and one's own body weight for resistance.

Let's face it: If you weigh 160 pounds and have a body shaped like a pear, you can lose twenty of those pounds and still look like a pear. You've lost weight, but the basic shape of your body hasn't changed. Remember what my trainer Davis said to me several years back: "Honey, if you want to change those thighs and those arms, you're gonna have to pump some iron!"? Well, now I'm telling you the same thing. No, I'm *not* suggesting that you have to go to the gym and bench-press 200 pounds or that you have to develop forearms the size of Mr. Olympia (unless that's your goal, of course). If you want to reshape the muscles that are situated on your skeletal frame, the only way is through weight training. Not only will weight training change your shape, it will also change your metabolism. Remember what I told you in Fat Facts: The more muscle (lean body mass) you have, the higher your metabolism and the more calories you burn. *Fantastic—I love that concept!*

In order for muscle to change (i.e., become firmer), it must be overloaded—pushed beyond its normal working capacity. To do this, you must use resistance tools (weights) and follow an organized program or training system. The Body Sculpting program is set up to be simple, practical, and easy to perform. In it you must perform a certain number of organized sets of exercises and repetitions. These are called "sets" and "reps." *Sets* are a predetermined grouping of exercises; for example, eight bicep curls performed one after the other (the number of reps) constitute a set of bicep curls. So if I say, "Do two sets of bicep curls," I'm asking you to do two sets of eight for a total of sixteen bicep curls, or sixteen reps. *Whatever exercise you're performing, the general rule is this: Stay between three to four sets of eight to twelve repetitions.*

Anatomy 101
Muscle . . . Use It or Lose It

Before you begin the Body Sculpting Workout, you should have some basic knowledge of the muscular system. Knowing the names of the muscles, where they're located, and how each one functions will make it easier for you to understand and translate the specific movements in the workout. Plus, the more you know about your body and how it works, the less likely you will be to waste your money on gimmicky exercise products that can't possibly give you the results that they promise.

Beginning from head to toe, let's look at the major muscles in your body and their primary function, which exercises are used to strengthen and build the muscles, plus the benefits you'll receive from working these particular muscles. (Also, for those of you who may become interested in further weight training once you outgrow your hand weights, I'll also provide you with the slang—"Gym Talk"—for each major muscle. Knowing "Gym Talk" is essential to fitting in once you make the big transition to the "serious" gyms.)

SHOULDER MUSCLES (DELTOIDS);
GYM TALK: DELTS

▲ FUNCTION: Lift arms to the side, assist other muscles in flexing, extending, and rotating arms.

▲ EXERCISES: Lateral raises, anterior raises, shoulder presses, reverse flys.

▲ BENEFITS: Broader shoulders make your hips appear narrower and your posture straighter. Stronger posterior (rear) shoulder muscles contribute to better posture.

CHEST MUSCLES (PECTORALS);
GYM TALK: PECS

▲ FUNCTION: Adduct arms (bring them together toward the center of the body), flex the humerus (upper arm bone) and rotate it inward.

▲ EXERCISES: Supine (on your back) chest presses, bench presses, flys, and push-ups.

▲ BENEFITS: A stronger chest contributes to good posture and gives a firmer-looking upper body.

UPPER BACK MUSCLES (RHOMBOIDS, TRAPEZIUS):
GYM TALK: TRAPS

▲ FUNCTION: Rotate scapula (shoulder blade), raise shoulders, adduct arms (bring them back down when they're lifted).

▲ EXERCISES: Shrugs, reverse flys, overhead presses.

▲ BENEFITS: Strengthen neck muscles that support the head more efficiently and reduce risk of potential neck injuries. Balance the appearance of the upper neck and shoulders. (Eliminate the "pencil-necked geek" look.)

BACK MUSCLES (LATISSIMUS DORSI);
GYM TALK: WINGS, LATS

▲ FUNCTION: Adduct arms (bring back down) and medially rotate the humerus (upper arm bone). This is the muscle group that helps you pull objects.

▲ EXERCISES: Lat pulldowns—front and back, seated rows, low rows, and single arm rows.

▲ BENEFITS: Wider lats make your waist appear narrower. They help improve your posture and increase your strength for pulling.

STOMACH MUSCLES, ABDOMEN (RECTUS
ABDOMINUS, INTERNAL AND EXTERNAL OBLIQUES);
GYM TALK: ABS, FINGERS (SERRATUS
ABDOMINALS)

▲ FUNCTION: Flex vertebrae, rotate trunk.

▲ EXERCISES: Crunches, rotation crunches, reverse crunches.

▲ BENEFITS: Support lower back, reduce low-back pain, contribute to good posture. (Underdeveloped abs don't look very good in a swimsuit. What you want are "washboard" abs—they look terrific in a bikini!)

MIDDLE-ARM MUSCLES (BICEPS);
GYM TALK: GUNS

▲ FUNCTION: Flex arm and forearm, bring hand toward shoulder. (These are your eating and drinking muscles, so watch out!)

▲ EXERCISES: Bicep curl variations, supine curls, isolation curls, barbell curls, reverse curls, hammer curls.

▲ BENEFITS: *Shapelier arms.* (Stronger biceps help you lift objects like heavy grocery bags and chubby toddlers.)

BACK-OF-ARM MUSCLES (TRICEPS);
GYM TALK: HORSESHOE (THAT'S THE SHAPE YOU
WANT YOUR TRICEP TO HAVE)

▲ FUNCTION: Extend the forearm, straighten a bent elbow. These are the muscles that help you push objects. (They're great to use when you're in one of those "all you can eat" restaurants: Use your triceps to push yourself away from the table!)

▲ EXERCISES: Tricep extensions—overhead and rear, French presses, dips.

▲ BENEFITS: Increase your ability to push heavy objects and eliminate the "flabby arm syndrome." (When you wave good-bye, does your tricep wave, too?)

UPPER FRONT LEG MUSCLES (QUADRICEPS);
GYM TALK: QUADS, QUADS WITH A SWEEP

▲ FUNCTION: Extend and flex the leg.

▲ EXERCISES: Leg extensions, leg presses, squats, pliés, lunges.

▲ BENEFITS: Stronger legs take the stress off your upper body and help prevent knee injuries.

BACK-OF-LEG MUSCLES (HAMSTRINGS, BICEP FEMORIS);
GYM TALK: HAMS

▲ FUNCTION: Flex the knee.

▲ EXERCISES: Hamstring curls, lunges, pliés, squats, leg presses.

▲ BENEFITS: Stronger, more flexible hamstrings help prevent knee injuries and alleviate undue muscle imbalance, which can create lower-back pain. (A well-developed hamstring should be round in the back of your leg, not the side of your leg. Did it all shift one day when you weren't looking?)

HIP MUSCLES (GLUTEUS MEDIUS);
GYM TALK: GLUTES

▲ FUNCTION: Abduct (move outward) and medially rotate the thigh. Lift leg to the side.

▲ EXERCISES: Side leg lifts.

▲ BENEFITS: Shapes the hips, tightens the glutes.

BUTTOCK MUSCLES (GLUTEUS MAXIMUS);
GYM TALK: GLUTES

▲ FUNCTION: Extend, abduct, and rotate thigh laterally. Lift legs to the back.

▲ EXERCISES: Squats, leg presses, lunges, pliés, hip extensions, rear attitudes. (Can a butt have an "attitude"? I know of a few . . .)

▲ BENEFITS: Tight, round, shapely, squeezable rear end. Need I say more?

CALF MUSCLES (GASTROCNEMIUS);

GYM TALK: DIAMONDS

- ▲ FUNCTION: Flex ankle and knee joints.
- ▲ EXERCISES: Toe raises, calf raises, heel lifts, high arch relevé, step training.
- ▲ BENEFITS: Shape lower leg and assist in ankle strength and stability.

Now you have the basic knowledge about your muscular system and which exercises will shape your muscles most effectively. Use this reference chart and the photographs on pages 212–213 throughout the initial learning phase of the Body Sculpting Workout. Now, get ready to pump that body!

What You'll Need

A variety of resistance tools exist on the market today—hand and leg weights, thick rubber bands, exercise tubing, and weight-training machines. For the sake of simplicity, I'll be demonstrating this workout using simple hand and leg weights, which can be purchased at any sporting-goods store. I also recommend purchasing a comfortable pair of weight gloves to wear so that your hands won't develop calluses.

How Heavy?

	▲ HAND WEIGHT	▲ LEG WEIGHT
▲ BEGINNER:	2–3 POUNDS	1–2 POUNDS
▲ INTERMEDIATE:	5–8 POUNDS	3–4 POUNDS
▲ ADVANCED:	8–12 POUNDS	5 POUNDS

As you progress and get stronger, increase weights in two-pound increments. The important thing to remember is to build up gradually. If you're overzealous and start off with heavy weights, your muscles will quickly become sore and you'll probably stop the program. Be patient: Michelangelo didn't carve his statues overnight; "chiseling" *your* muscles takes time, too.

Which Tunes?

The music that I use for this workout has approximately 130 to 134 beats per minute—a tempo that's fast enough to elevate your heart rate but not so slow that it puts you to sleep.

Keep It Safe!

1. Consult your physician before beginning this or any exercise program. Do not participate in any weight-training program without therapeutic approval or prescription from a physical therapist if you have any of the following conditions: hypertension, arthritis, bursitis, tendinitis, or muscular or orthopedic injuries.
2. Weight-train with proper footwear. Aerobic dance or crosstraining shoes work best. They provide both the cushioning and lateral support needed for squats and pliés.
3. Wear comfortable, nonrestrictive clothing.
4. Warm up and stretch before you use weights. Muscles and joints become tight from resistance training. Stretching will help maintain your flexibility.
5. Don't hyperextend (straighten beyond your normal range) joints while lifting weights.

6. Don't swing the weights; control each movement. When you're lifting weights above your head, don't bring them back down too quickly. Always lower them slowly and gently.

7. Don't just squeeze at the top end or the bottom end of the move—work the muscles through a full range of motion.

8. Refer frequently to the body alignment in each of the photos to ensure that your body is in proper alignment.
   Body Alignment Techniques:

   - Stand tall
   - Keep shoulders aligned over hips
   - Keep pelvis tilted when appropriate
   - Keep neck neutral, not tilted back or forward
   - Keep abdominals tight
   - Do not arch the back

9. Never hold your breath! *Exhale* on the effort (the hardest part of the move); *inhale* while returning to the starting position.

10. Work progressively—focus on the larger muscle groups first and then work on the smaller groups. Example:

▲ LARGE MUSCLE GROUP	▲ SMALL MUSCLE GROUP
Legs	Biceps
Gluteals	Triceps
Chest	Abdominals
Back	Shoulders

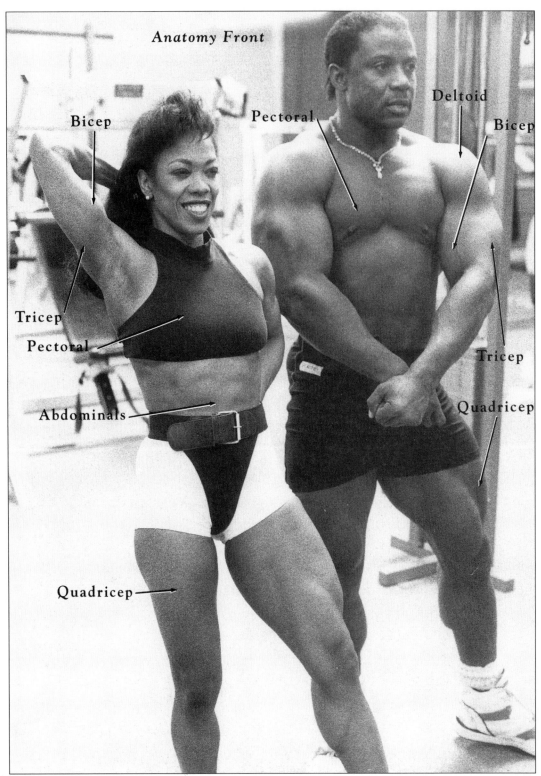

Anatomy Front

Bicep

Pectoral

Deltoid

Bicep

Tricep

Pectoral

Abdominals

Tricep

Quadricep

Quadricep

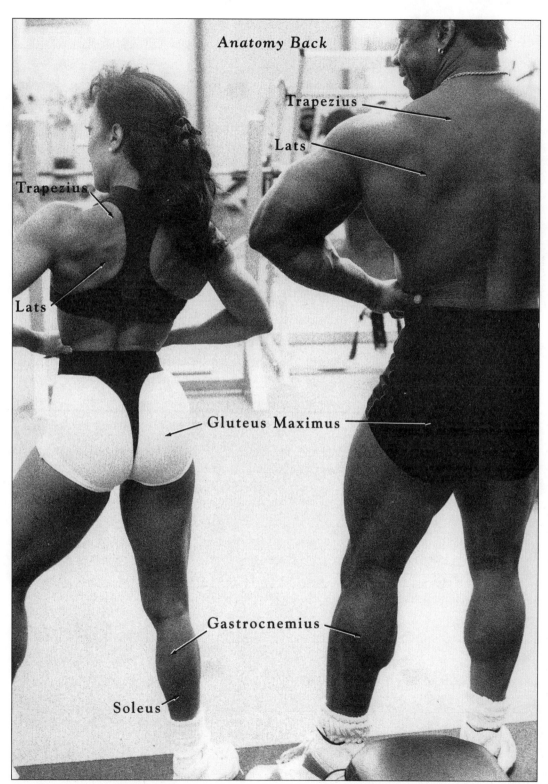

Anatomy Back

Trapezius

Lats

Trapezius

Lats

Gluteus Maximus

Gastrocnemius

Soleus

11. Work your body to create muscle *balance*. If you work your back, then also work your chest. If you're pressed for time, this can be done on separate days; just don't totally neglect a certain muscle or group of muscles. Men tend to pump up their pecs and forget their legs—and many end up looking like balloons! Then there are the women who do leg lifts until they're blue in the face: They end up with hip bursitis and triceps that jiggle when they wave.

12. Rest thirty seconds to one minute between sets—no longer.

13. You should rest a muscle group forty-eight hours before working it again with resistance.

14. If you choose to work with leg weights, don't use them during movements that travel. Use them only with stationary, isolation movements.

15. Be cautious at all times: Safety first, challenge second. Don't push yourself to the point of injury.

16. Keep your body hydrated. Drink plenty of water before, during, and after your workout.

17. Cool down gradually and stretch.

Chapter Eleven:
Movements and Patterns

Strength is not just mental . . . it is physical.

Have you looked at yourself naked in a mirror lately and seen a part of your body you wish you could change? If the answer is yes, then you need this section. The words "body sculpting" speak for themselves. You can do aerobic activity until you drop and still not change the shape of your body. If you want to have a balanced physique, you must lift weights. Just think how wonderful it would be if you had perfectly sculpted shoulders and you'd never have to wear another pair of shoulder pads. Not only would your figure improve but your physical carriage would project power and strength.

Breaking it down into body parts:

Legs:

Basic Lunge with Bicep Curl

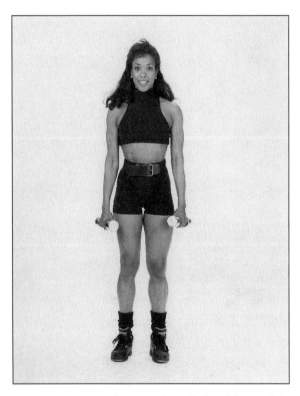

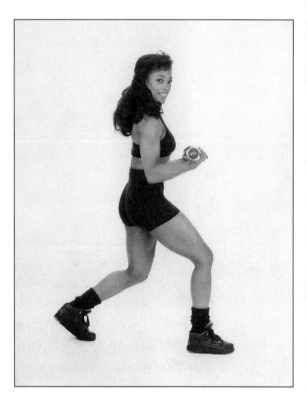

1. Arms to side, knees relaxed shoulder width apart, pelvis neutral.

2. Left leg steps forward, knee tracking over ankle, weight over hips with emphasis on heel, elbows to side, palms curl toward chest.

Bring left leg back to starting position and repeat on right.

Single Leg Lunge
(using chair)

Squat

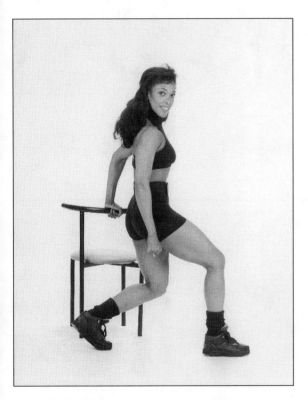

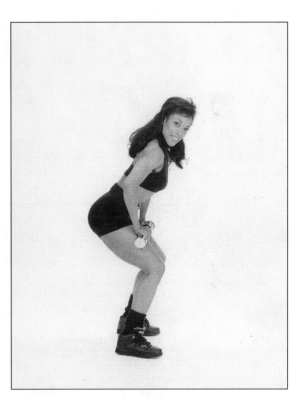

1. Right hand on chair, left leg steps forward, knee tracking over ankle, weight over hips, elbows to side, palms curl toward chest.

Bring left leg back to starting position and repeat.

Turn and repeat movement on right leg with left hand on chair.

1. With light weights resting on thighs (or shoulders), squat to a sitting position for a count of two. Pelvis is neutral, shoulders neutral, weight over heels. On the way up squeeze buttocks and press through heels.

Squat with Side Leg Lift

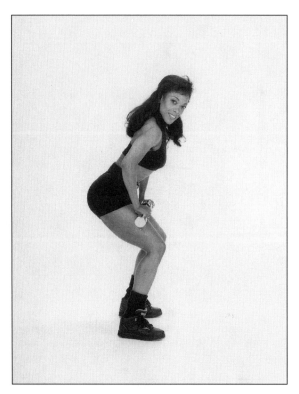 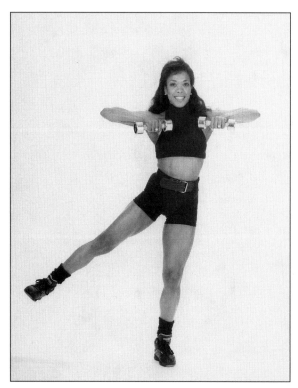

1. With light weights resting on thighs (or shoulders), squat to a sitting position for a count of two. Pelvis is neutral, shoulders neutral, weight over heels.

2. On the way up squeeze buttocks and abduct (extend) left leg to side, raise elbows in an upright row, wrists neutral.

Return left leg to starting squat position and repeat on right side.

Squat with Chair

Squat with Hamstring Curl

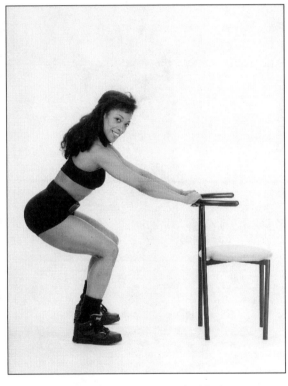

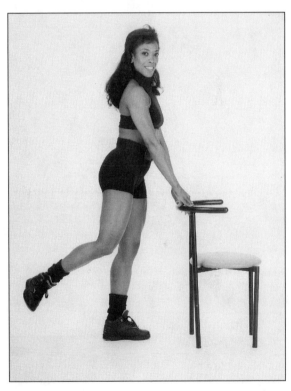

1. Stand facing back of chair, hold chair at top, and squat to a sitting position for a count of two. Pelvis is neutral, shoulders neutral, weight over heels. On the way up, squeeze buttocks and press through heels.

1. Stand facing back of chair, hold chair at top and squat to a sitting position for a count of two. Pelvis is neutral, shoulders neutral, weight over heels. On the way up, squeeze left buttock and curl left leg behind body, tightening heel and contracting hamstring (or squeezing back of leg).

Return to squat postion and repeat right leg.

Abductors

Abductors with Chair

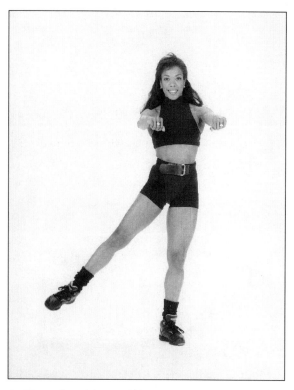

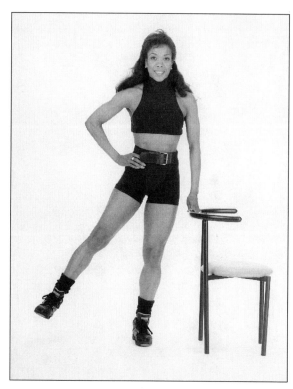

1. Feet shoulder-width apart, lift left leg, foot flexed and tighten through hip as you lift. Raise arms forward, palms facing floor.

Bring foot back to starting position and repeat.

1. Feet shoulder-width apart, lift left leg, foot flexed and tighten through hip as you lift. Bring foot back to starting position and repeat.

(For adduction [inner thigh] simply lead with heel and cross center line of body toward chair.)

Hip Extension with Chair

1. Feet shoulder-width apart, squeeze buttocks and extend leg to back, hands resting on back of chair. Point toe as you lift and repeat on other side.

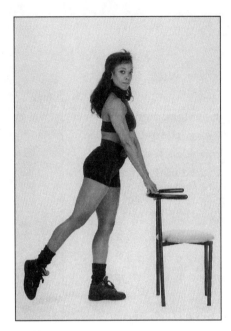

Leg Extension with Chair

1. Seated with hands on armrest, extend left leg forward squeezing through top of thighs (quadriceps), toe pointed—4 counts on the way up and 2 counts on the way down. Repeat on right.

2. Repeat same sequence with foot flexed.

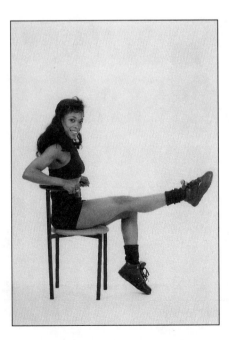

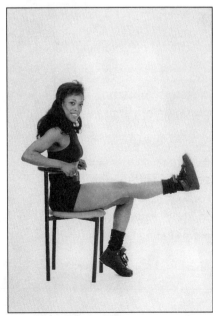

Pliés with Weights

1. Natural turnout from hips with heels together, shoulders back, pelvis tucked under, hands at top of thighs holding light hand weights.

2. Step open to second position maintaining turnout. Lift left arm to upright position, palms facing floor.

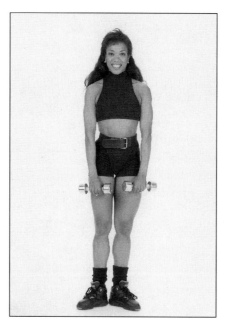
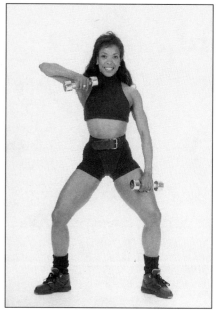

3. Return to starting postion, both arms go down.

4. Step open to second position maintaining turnout. Lift both arms to upright position, palms facing floor.

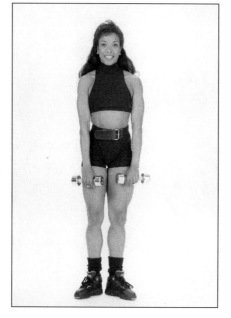
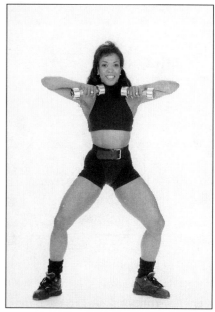

Abductors on Floor #1

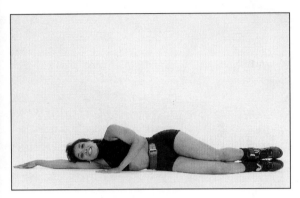

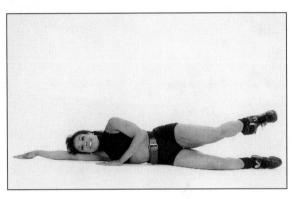

1. Lie flat on side, head resting on arm, cervical spine neutral, both knees slightly bent, abdominal wall contracted, knees together, right hand on floor supporting position.

2. Lift right leg 12 to 18 inches, contracting through hips.

Abductors on Floor #2

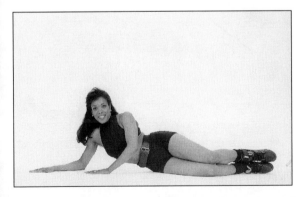

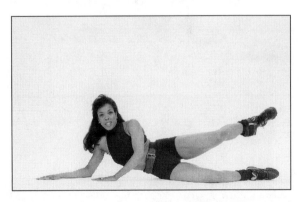

1. Left arm is bent, resting on elbow (avoid rolling onto shoulder, maintain shoulder stability), cervical spine neutral, both knees slightly bent, abdominal wall contracted, knees together, right hand on floor supporting position.

2. Lift right leg 12 to 18 inches, contracting through hips.

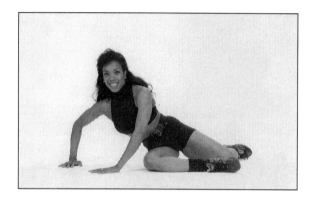

Abductors with Rear Attitude

1. Both arms are forward, resting on hands. Legs in rear attitude position with right knee on floor, right foot (rear foot) flexed. Cervical spine neutral, both knees bent, abdominal wall contracted.

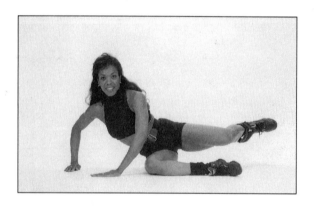

2. Lift right leg parallel to right hip, contract through hips.

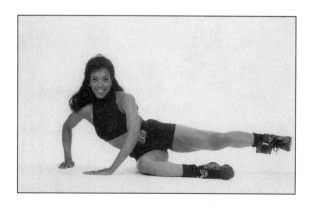

3. Return to #1.

4. Lift right leg in straight position, parallel to right hip, contract through hips.

Hamstring Curl
(flat on stomach or on knees)

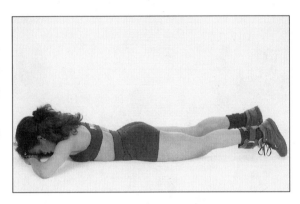

1. Flat on stomach, head down on hands, legs relaxed.

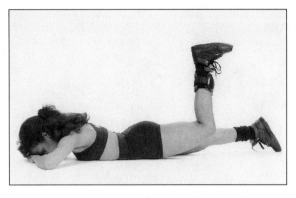

2. Squeeze buttocks, bend right knee with heel moving toward buttock, foot flexed. Return to position.

(or)

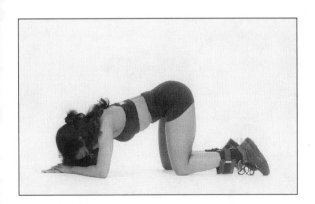

1. Support weight on elbows, head down on hands, abdominals contracted, pelvis tucked under.

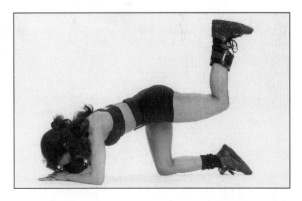

2. Squeeze buttocks, bend right knee with heel moving toward buttock, foot flexed. Repeat opposite leg.

Rear Leg Lift

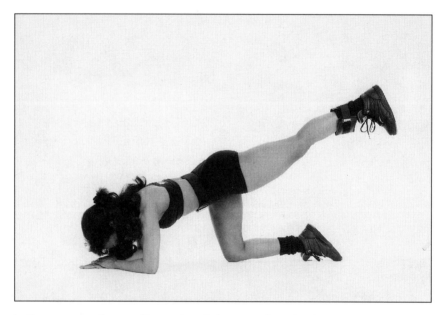

1. Support weight on elbows, head down on hands, abdominals contracted, pelvis tucked under.

2. Squeeze buttocks, lift left leg with heel flexed. Return to position #1. Repeat opposite leg.

Upper Body:

BICEPS

Peak Curls with Crossovers

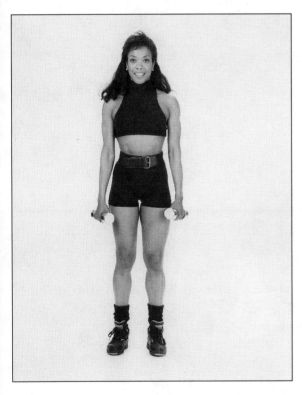 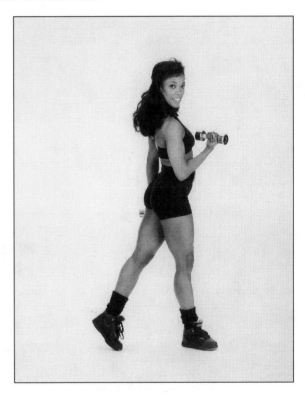

1. Starting postion: first position turnout, palms to thighs.

2. Left leg crosses over right, left arm curls with palm toward shoulder.

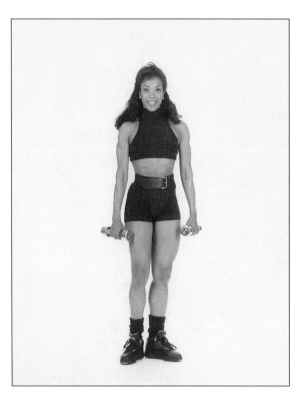

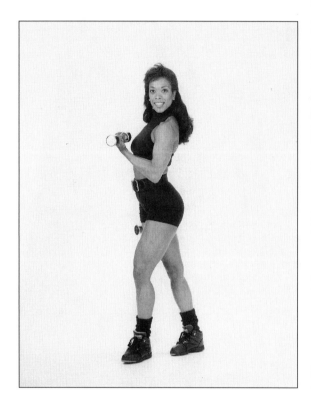

3. Return to starting position.

4. Repeat #2 on right side.

Hammer Curls

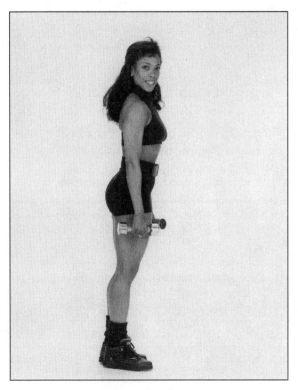

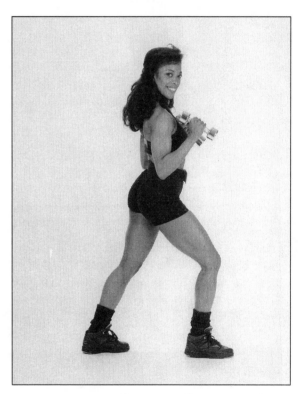

1. Starting position: natural turnout in first position, weights against thighs.

2. Lunge forward with left leg. As arms curl, palms face each other with weights lifting to top of shoulder.

Return to #1 and repeat.

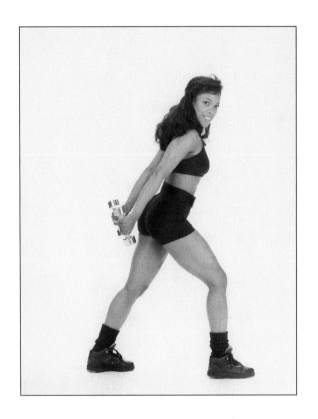

TRICEPS

Double Extension

1. Starting position: natural turnout in first position, weights against thighs.

SEE HAMMER CURL 1.

2. Lunge forward with left leg, both palms extend to back (facing each other), squeezing triceps.

Return to #1 and repeat.

Overhead Extension

1. Legs in second position, pelvis tucked under, arm above head, elbow bent with weight in hand.

2. Extend elbow, straightening arm above head.

Return to #1 and repeat.

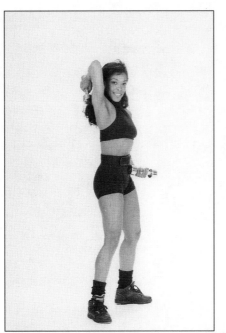
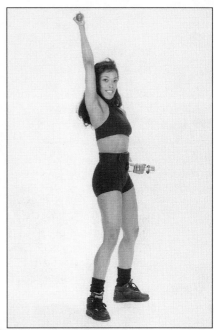

Press Down

1. Left knee bent, left toe pointed, weights in bicep curl position, palms toward chest.

2. Step across body with left leg, extend arms in front of body, palms facing thighs, contract triceps.

Return to #1 and repeat.

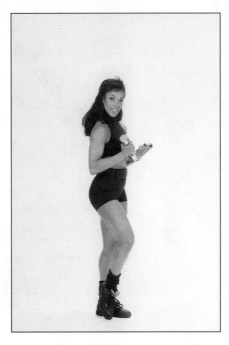
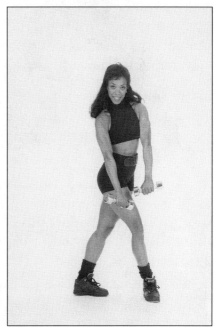

Lats:

Single Rows

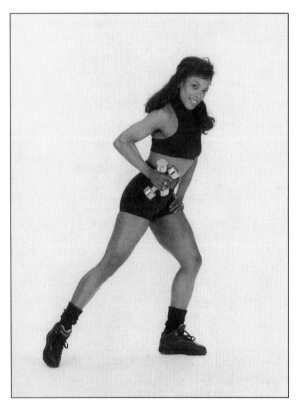 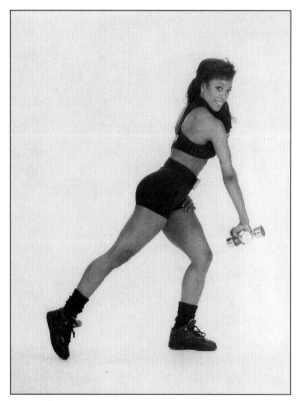

1. Right leg turns out to right, left leg out to side, toe pointed. With both weights in left hand, elbow close to body, palm facing hip, shoulders relaxed.

2. Rotate body forward, pressing weights toward floor and release upper back.

Return to #1, contracting lats on way back. Repeat and then switch to opposite side.

Single Rows with Rear Leg Extension

1. Right leg turns out to right, left leg out to side, toe pointed. With both weights in left hand, elbow close to body, palm facing hip, shoulders relaxed. (See starting position for Single Row)

2. Rotate body forward, lift left leg to rear with toe pointed (do not arch back), pressing weights toward floor and release upper back.

Return to #1, contracting lats on way back. Repeat and then switch to opposite side.

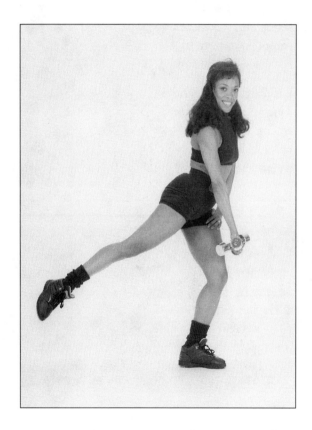

Double Rows

1. Begin in squat position, feet shoulder-width apart, pelvis neutral, shoulders relaxed, arms extended to front of body at 45-degree angle.

2. Straighten knees, squeeze buttocks, contract upper back, elbows come behind spine with weights facing hips.

Repeat.

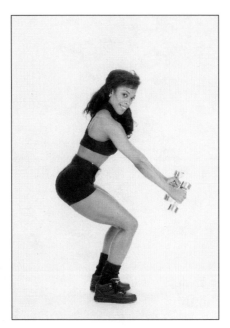
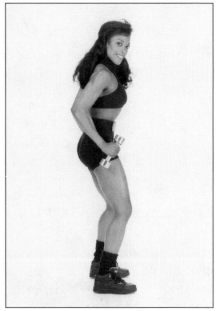

Reverse Flys

1. Begin in squat position, feet shoulder-width apart, pelvis neutral, shoulders relaxed, arms extended to front of body at 45-degree angle.

2. Straighten knees, squeeze buttocks, contract upper back, elbows come behind spine with palms facing down.

Repeat.

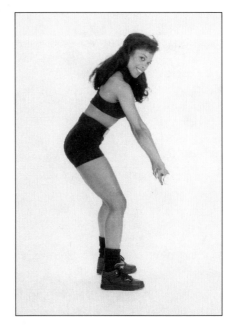
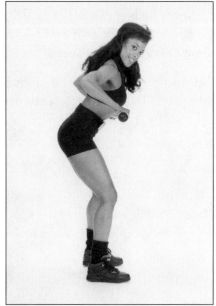

Military Press

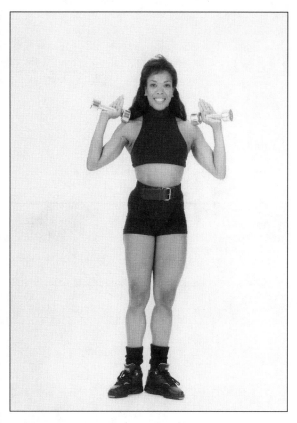

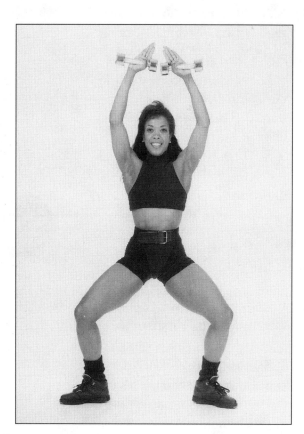

1. Start in first-position turnout, palms at shoulders facing forward.

2. Plié and press palms overhead.

Push-ups:

Regular Push-ups

1. Starting position: arms shoulder-width apart, fingers forward, elbows slightly bent, abdominals contracted, pelvis tucked, knees bent.

2. Lower chest to floor, elbows to outside, abdominals remain contracted. Return to #1, contracting chest as you straighten arms.

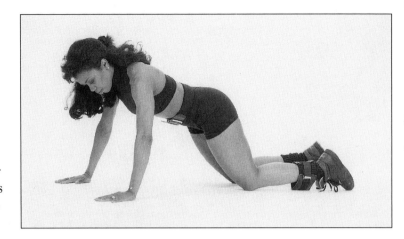

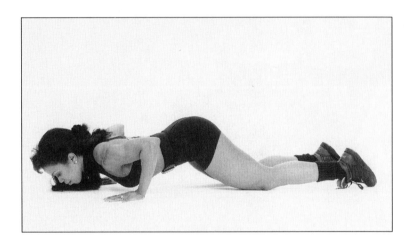

Triceps Push-ups

1. Starting position: flat on floor, palms are next to chest, arms shoulder-width apart, fingers forward, elbows bent behind spine, abdominals contracted, pelvis tucked, knees bent.

2. Straighten elbows and lift body weight, contracting chest as you straighten arms. Return to #1 maintaining bent-elbow position. See Regular Push-up.

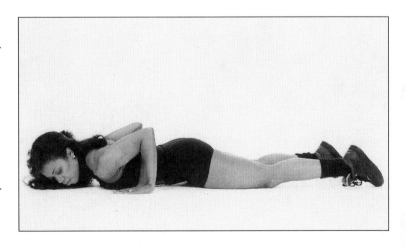

Safety Tips:

1. Keep the lower back neutral.
2. Inhale through the nose. Exhale through the mouth.
3. Keep the contraction constant throughout the entire range of motion during crunch movement.
4. Keep abdominals contracted (tight) at all times.
5. Do not pull on the head or strain the neck during crunches.
6. Keep the cervical spine neutral at all times.
7. Don't arch the lower back during crunches.

Abdominals:

Basic Crunch

1. Knees bent, pelvis tucked, back neutral, head on floor. Place hand on lower abdominal wall to establish posterior pelvis tilt.

2. Palms together, pressing toward knees and lift chest forward raising shoulder blades off floor and contracting through abdominals. Hold each set for 4 counts.

Return to #1 and repeat.

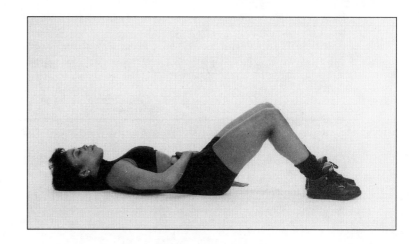

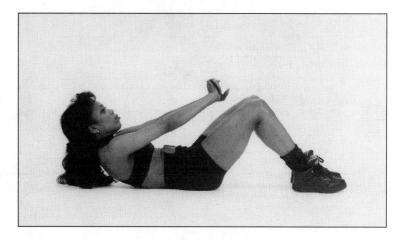

Rotation Crunch

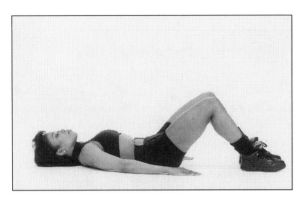

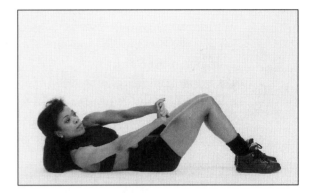

1. Knees bent, both arms flat on floor, pelvis tucked, back neutral, head on floor.

2. Rotate upper body up and across to left with both arms pressing toward left side.

Return to #1 and repeat on right side.

Oblique Crossover

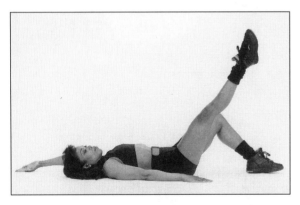

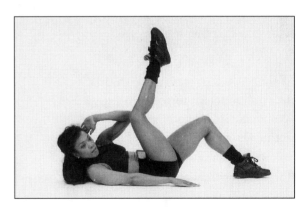

1. One knee is bent, the other is straight; one arm is extended over head, the other remains on floor. Pelvis tucked, back neutral, head on floor.

2. Lift right arm to cross body, left leg bends and meets elbow at center of body.

Reverse Crunch—Knee to Chest

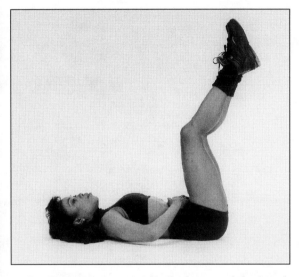 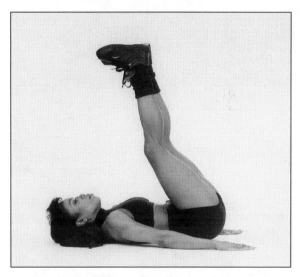

1. Starting position: on back, legs are lifted with knees slightly bent, hands on lower abdominals to establish pelvis tilt.

2. Hands to sides by hips, feet flexed, contract abdominals and lift buttocks one inch off floor. Hold for 2 counts and return to floor.

Oblique Reverse Crossover

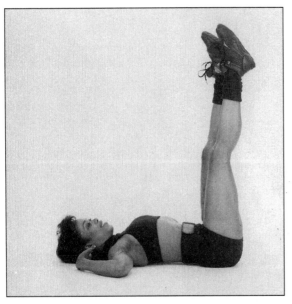

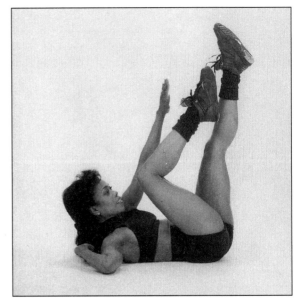

1. Lie on back, hands by head, toes pointed, posterior pelvic tilt.

2. Left knee bends to chest, right arm reaches across body with trunk rotation and toward left foot.

Return to #1 and repeat on opposite side.

Rollback Level #1

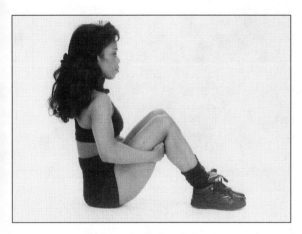

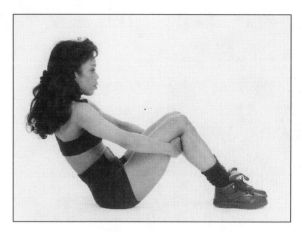

1. Sit upright, hands behind legs for support, feet flat on floor.

2. Chest crunches toward thighs to form a "C" position. (Don't arch back.)

Rollback Level #2

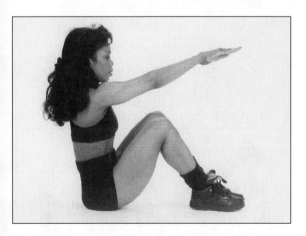

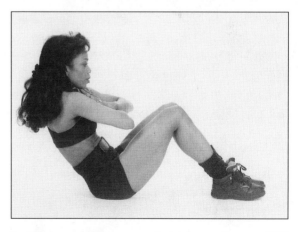

1. Sit upright, extend in front of body, feet flat on floor.

2. Chest crunches toward thighs to form a "C" position, arms cross chest. (Don't arch back.)

Return to #1.

241

Obliques Rollback Level #2

1. Sit upright, extend arms in front of body, feet flat on floor. (See #1, Rollback Level #1.)

2. Roll back and crunch with rotation to left, arms also rotate left.

Return to #1 and repeat to right.

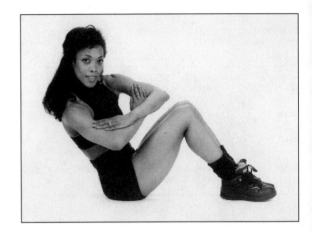

Oblique Crunch

1. Lie on left side, both knees facing left, head toward ceiling, chest rotated to ceiling.

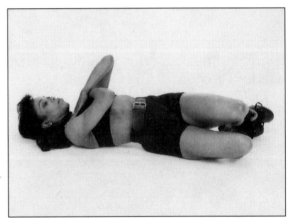

2. Roll and crunch arms reaching toward right, chest and head to ceiling.
Return to #1 and repeat to left.

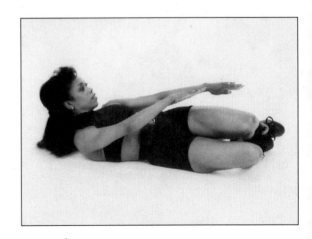

Chapter Twelve:
Body Sculpting Workouts

Level 1 — Beginner

If you are new to working out, remember to work at a moderate level with light weights (two to three pounds) and low repetitions (two sets of eight). Several of the standing sculpting moves outlined in the workout allow you to support yourself with a chair to help you maintain your balance and proper alignment. Your outlined workout provides you with time lines to follow:

Warm-up preparation and stretch: 8 to 10 minutes
Body sculpting workout: 15 minutes standing, 10 minutes floor work
Cool-down and flexibility stretch: 8 to 10 minutes

Level 2 — Intermediate

If you are familiar with exercise and have been involved in some type of aerobic conditioning and body-sculpting workouts for more than three months, it's fine to work with heavier hand weights (three to five pounds) and higher repetitions (three sets of eight to twelve). Your workout is coordinated as follows:

Warm-up preparation and stretch: 8 to 10 minutes
Body sculpting workout: 20 minutes standing, 10 minutes floor work
Cool-down and flexibility stretch: 10 minutes

Level 3 — Advanced

If you have been involved in aerobic conditioning for six months or more, you are ready to challenge yourself with heavier weights (five to seven pounds) and higher repetitions (four sets of eight to twelve). As you become familiar with the moves, you can add more variations that you feel comfortable with.

Warm-up preparation and stretch: 8 to 10 minutes
Body sculpting workout: 30 minutes standing, 15 minutes floor work
Cool-down and flexibility stretch: 10 minutes

Beginner — Intermediate — Advanced
Body Sculpting Workout Outline

(Total Minutes: 45 to 65)

Warm-up preparation and stretch: 8 to 10 minutes
Repeat each movement 8 to 16 times.
(See Chapter Six for movement descriptions.)

Deep Breathing
Pelvic Tilt
Pelvic Tilt with Spine Isolation
Shoulder Rotation
Shoulder Rolls
Torso Isolations

JAZZ ISOLATION SERIES

Rib-Cage Isolation
Hip Isolation
Chest Cross
Parallel Passé
Bicep Curl/Hip Isolation

STATIC ISOLATION STRETCH

Runner's Lunge
Calf Stretch
Hamstring Isolation
Groin Isolation
Posterior Shoulder Stretch
Anterior Shoulder Stretch
Head Tilt
Chin to Chest

Beginner Workout

1. Single leg lunge using chair (2 sets of 8 each leg)
   Time elapsed: 2 minutes
2. Squat with chair (2 sets of 8)
   Time elapsed: 3 minutes

3. Squat with hamstring curl (2 sets of 8 each leg)
   Time elapsed: 5 minutes
4. Abductors with chair (2 sets of 8 each leg)
   Time elapsed: 7 minutes
5. Hip extension with chair (2 sets of 8 each leg)
   Time elapsed: 9 minutes
6. Leg extension with chair (2 sets of 8 each leg)
   Time elapsed: 11 minutes
7. Bicep peak curls with crossovers (2 sets of 8 each leg)
   Time elapsed: 13 minutes
8. Tricep double extension (2 sets of 8)
   Time elapsed: 14 minutes
9. Single rows (2 sets of 8)
   Time elapsed: 15 minutes
10. Double rows (2 sets of 8)
    Time elapsed: 16 minutes

GO TO FLOOR:

11. Regular push-ups (2 sets of 8)
12. Tricep push-ups (2 sets of 8)

ABDOMINALS:

13. Basic crunch (3 sets of 8)
14. Rotation crunch (3 sets of 8)
15. Oblique crossover (3 sets of 8)
16. Reverse crunch (3 sets of 8)
    Time elapsed: 25 minutes (Beginner workout complete; continue with cool-down movements.)

Intermediate-to-Advanced Workout

1. Basic lunge with bicep curl (intermediate — 2 sets of 10 each leg; advanced — 3 sets of 8 to 12 each leg)
   Intermediate time elapsed: 2.5 minutes
   Advanced time elapsed: 3 minutes

2. Squat (intermediate — 2 sets of 10; advanced — 3 sets of 8 to 12)
   Intermediate time elapsed: 4.5 minutes
   Advanced time elapsed: 6 minutes

3. Squat with side leg lift (intermediate — 2 sets of 10 each leg; advanced — 3 sets of 8 to 12 each leg)
   Intermediate time elapsed: 7 minutes
   Advanced time elapsed: 9 minutes

4. Squat with hamstring curl (intermediate — 2 sets of 10 each leg; advanced — 3 sets of 8 to 12 each leg)
   Intermediate time elapsed: 9.5 minutes
   Advanced time elapsed: 11 minutes

5. Abductors (intermediate — 2 sets of 10 each leg; advanced — 3 sets of 8 to 12 each leg)
   Intermediate time elapsed: 12 minutes
   Advanced time elapsed: 14 minutes

6. Pliés with weights (intermediate — 2 sets of 10; advanced — 3 sets of 8 to 12)
   Intermediate time elapsed: 14.5 minutes (Move directly to triceps.)
   Advanced time elapsed: 17 minutes

Upper Body:

7. Bicep peak curls with crossovers (advanced — 3 sets of 8 to 12)
Advanced time elapsed: 20 minutes

8. Hammer curls (advanced — 3 sets of 8 to 12)
Advanced time elapsed: 22 minutes

9. Tricep double extension (intermediate — 2 sets of 10; advanced — 3 sets of 8 to 12)
Intermediate time elapsed: 16.5 minutes (Move directly to lats.)
Advanced time elapsed: 25 minutes

10. Tricep overhead extension (advanced — 3 sets of 8 to 12)
Advanced time elapsed: 27.5 minutes

11. Tricep press down (advanced — 3 sets of 8 to 12)
Advanced time elapsed: 30 minutes

Lats:

12. Single rows (intermediate — 2 sets of 10; advanced — 3 sets of 8 to12)
Intermediate time elapsed: 18 minutes
Advanced time elapsed: 32 minutes

13. Single rows with rear leg extension (intermediate — 2 sets of 10; advanced — 3 sets of 8 to 12)
Intermediate time elapsed: 20 minutes
Advanced time elapsed: 34 minutes

Go to Floor:

14. Abductors on floor #1 (intermediate — 2 sets of 10; advanced — 3 sets of 8 to 12)

Intermediate time elapsed: 22 minutes
Advanced time elapsed: 36.5 minutes

15. Abductors on floor #2 (advanced only — 3 sets of 8 to 12)

    Advanced time elapsed: 22.5 minutes

16. Abductors with rear attitude (intermediate — 2 sets of 10; advanced — 3 sets of 12)

    Intermediate time elapsed: 24 minutes
    Advanced time elapsed: 39 minutes

17. Regular push-ups (intermediate — 2 sets of 10; advanced — 3 sets of 12)

    Intermediate time elapsed: 24 minutes
    Advanced time elapsed: 39 minutes

18. Tricep push-ups (intermediate — 2 sets of 10; advanced — 3 sets of 12)

    Intermediate time elapsed: 26 minutes
    Advanced time elapsed: 41 minutes

ABDOMINALS:

19. Basic crunch (3 sets of 10)
20. Rotation crunch (3 sets of 10)
21. Oblique crossover (3 sets of 10)
22. Reverse crunch (3 sets of 10)
23. Oblique reverse crossover (3 sets of 10)
24. Rollback level #1 (3 sets of 10)
25. Rollback level #2 (3 sets of 10)
26. Oblique rollback level #2 (3 sets of 10)

    Intermediate time elapsed: 36 minutes
    Advanced time elapsed: 50 minutes

COOL-DOWN:

Inverted Hurdler Stretch
Front and Rear Attitude Stretch
Second Position Dancer's Stretch
Crossover
Hamstring Stretch on Floor
Calf Stretch
Hamstring Isolation
Groin Isolation

Final note: This workout does not include all the moves outlined in "Pump That Body," Chapter Ten. As you become familiar with the workouts, simply add moves and take others out.

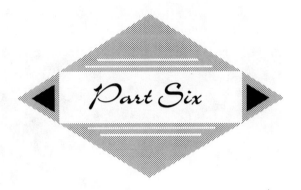

Part Six

DANCE, DANCE, DANCE—
THE TECHNIFUNK™
DANCE WORKOUT SERIES

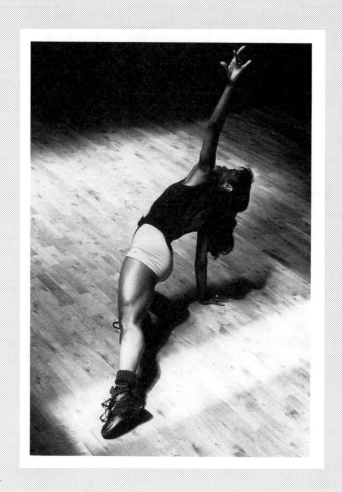

Chapter Thirteen:
The Future of Fitness

Dance, Dance, Dance

Ever since I was a little girl I've wanted to be a dancer, and for two years I did dance professionally with a jazz and African dance troupe. In hot pursuit of larger, more prestigious dance troupes, I discovered that none of them would hire me because I was "too short." I was destroyed: I thought my lifelong dream would never come true. Fortunately I was also involved in aerobics at the time, so the transition from professional dancer to professional aerobics instructor was a relatively smooth one. Since then I have always maintained a connection between my dance training and my aerobic dance training.

As a dancer, I was taught the principles of *balance, energy, and strength* and how they all pertain to *dance movement*—all of which come from the core or center of your body, from your heart and from your soul. When you're dancing, being *balanced* means you're able to go in many directions without falling and losing your focus. The same is true in any life situation. I felt it was important to integrate this basic philosophy regarding balance and centering into the mainstream of aerobics as well—that is why dance is such an important element in all my workouts.

Dance takes many forms; one of the latest is *funk*. Funk is the craze that's burning holes in soles (and souls) across the nation—in aerobic dance studios, health clubs, and community rec centers. A spin-off of MTV rap and dance group videos, funk was actually inspired by African tribal movements and contemporary jazz dance. Funk movements rely on the downbeat in music; they're lower to the ground (grounded), and upper-body isolations and stylized accents dominate the steps (e.g., Roger Rabbit, Troop, Run'n Man). Since funky rap music has become an official category in the Grammy Awards, there's no doubt in my mind that funk is here to stay. For me this translates into dozens of new funk moves we can learn.

For nondancers, however, funk movements are often too difficult and complex. To make it easier for my students to learn, I simplified the movements and added more traditional dance technique to come up with my own version: *Technifunk*™.

What Is Technifunk™?

Have there ever been days when you've said to yourself after an aerobics class, "If I do one more knee lift or jumping jack I'm going to scream! I'm so sick of this stuff!" Well, about four years ago, after teaching nothing but high-impact aerobics, that was exactly how I felt, too. I'd been teaching aerobics for more than thirteen years, and I'd finally gotten bored and frustrated with the old knee lifts and jumping jacks, the fast-paced bouncing and leaping around the aerobics room. It seemed to me that over the years aerobics had become a repetitive, kamikaze high-impact event lacking in any feeling whatsoever. In an effort to revitalize my classes and bring some of the *fun* back into aerobics again, I started to reincorporate dance-based moves that were lower impact, more expressive, more grounded, rhythmic, and fluid. The result was a program consisting of power moves and locomotion (across the floor) combinations. In the beginning I called it Cardio Power Funk. Today it has evolved into a program that combines traditional movement and dance techniques (e.g., ballet, jazz, and modern dance), MTV funk, and stylized aerobic power moves. I call it Technifunk™.

I decided on this combination for several reasons. First, dance technique gives your body wonderful, strong lines and forces work to take place from the center (which ultimately creates a sense of inner balance). Second, MTV funk allows you to be creative and expressive, to feel and explore movement—not to mention that it's a lot of fun! Last, I include aerobic power leg movements into the Technifunk™ workout primarily for intensity and to allow you to work the major muscles in your body. The more major muscles you use, the more aerobic a workout becomes. Plus, these power moves are great for firming up your lower body—they tighten your buns, shape your hips, and strengthen your abdominals.

Not only are *my* students excited and challenged by this new form of aerobic dance, but the thousands of instructors I've taught this program to say *their* students love it, too. One thing I'm always quick to point out to students and instructors is that there's really no "perfect" way to do Technifunk™. After you've learned the basic movements, much of the interpretation is left up to you—and that's where the freedom and the fun begin! Technifunk™ allows you to have a good time and to experiment, to personalize your workout (even though you may be in a class situation) and add your own special flair. Think of it as *aerobics with an attitude!*

A rhythm-impaired warning: We all go through many stages when we learn something new—especially with dance moves! The first stage is usually denial: "I'll *never* move like that—I have *no* sense of rhythm," or "She can move like that because she's small and she's a dancer!" *Don't talk yourself into giving up.* My students come in all shapes and sizes; some have had previous dance experience, but most have not. The point is they're *all* doing Technifunk™—and loving it! So c'mon, now—lace up those dancin' shoes! It's time to *move!*

What You'll Need

You don't need much to do Technifunk™. A wood-surfaced floor is preferable, but carpet is okay, too—just be careful. Oh yes, and you gotta have music. . . .

Which Tunes?

The Technifunk™ Dance Workout works best with funky, rap tunes. Slower (approximately 118–130 beats per minute) "house" or "hip-hop" music, or certain pop tunes work best for this workout.

Ask someone at your record store to recommend some music. I've made up my own tapes, which include songs from the following: Hammer, Heavy D, D.J. Jazzy Jeff, Janet Jackson, L. L. Cool J., and C & C Music Factory.

Keep It Safe!

Don't forget that Technifunk™ is different from traditional aerobics. The moves are more grounded, with a focus on upper-body and hip movements.

1. Consult your physician before beginning this or any exercise program.
2. Exercise with proper footwear, such as a light pair of aerobic dance shoes. (Don't wear the fashionable heavy boots for long periods of time—you could easily be injured.)
3. Wear comfortable loose clothing, or for more support try cotton Lycra tights and crop tops.
4. Warm up before your Technifunk™ Workout: Isolate the neck, shoulders, upper torso, rib cage, ankles, and calves.
5. During the first three to five minutes of precardio (that is, *before* maximum sweat time), concentrate on movements that travel front and back in order to give the knees and ankles more time to

warm up before initiating lateral movement.

6. When marching, don't bend at the waist because it creates too much stress on the lower back. Keep your abdominals tight, pelvis tucked under, shoulders back, and chest lifted.

7. Practice your dancer's turnout. External rotation should initiate from the hips in order to protect the knees; keep your knees tracking over your toes at all times.

8. When performing combinations and complicated movements, always *keep moving*. The tendency is to stop moving in order to learn the various movements. Develop ways of maintaining an aerobic heart rate or a consistent RPE level through marching or traveling as you make your transitions from one move to the next.

9. Keep your body hydrated. Drink plenty of water before, during, and after your workout.

10. Cool down gradually and stretch.

Chapter Fourteen:
Movements and Patterns

Dancing frees your soul.

We've all had bad days when we just want to get away from it all. A great way to escape is to dance. Once the music fills your body you forget whatever is going on in your life. Dancing creates powerful emotions. It breaks down inhibitions with each step. It is fun, inspirational, and the perfect way to feel good while you're getting in shape. Dancing not only makes you feel good, it makes you look good. It gives your body long, graceful lines and inspires you to greater heights of physical and emotional awareness. This is why dance is now being taught to physically impaired children across the United States.

Proper March

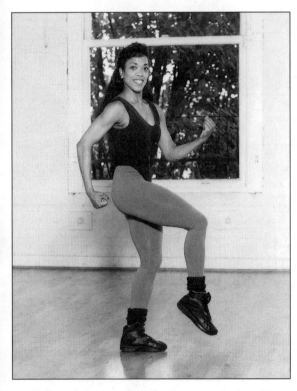

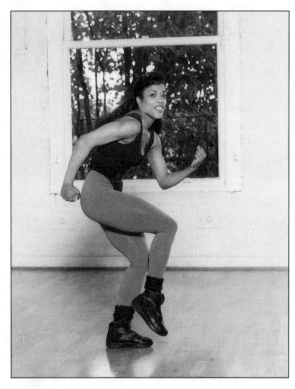

1. Right: Pelvis tucked, chest and shoulders upright, elbows bent. Begin your march on downbeat. Land toe, ball of foot, then heel.

2. Wrong: don't bend at the waist; don't hyper-extend your neck.

Funky Grapevine

1. Feet together, shoulders back, arms out to sides.

2. Step open with right leg, raise arms above head, hands in fist position.

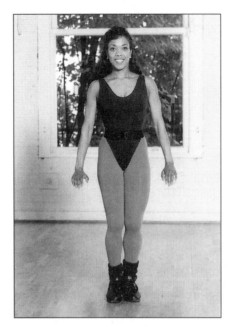
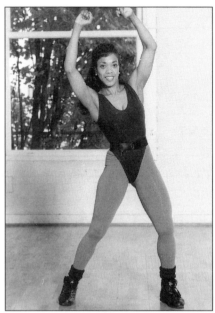

3. Cross left leg behind right, raise arms laterally with palms pressed out.

4. Repeat # 2.

5. Bring left leg in to meet right with left knee slightly bent.

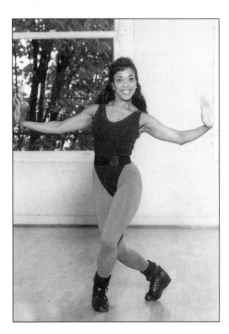
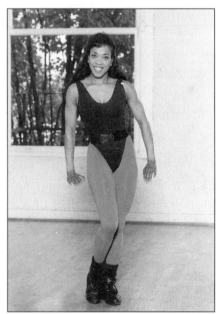

Wide Step

1. Start with both feet together in first position — jazz hands over abdominals.

2. Left foot steps out — left arm extends at angle above head.

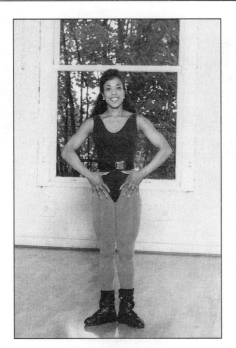
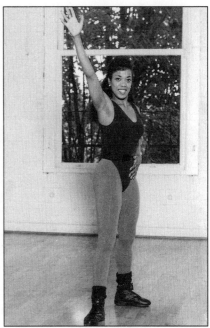

3. Right foot steps out — right arm extends out.

4. Left foot in — hand returns to abdominals.

5. Right foot in — hand returns to abdominals.

Return to # 1.

Total counts: 4

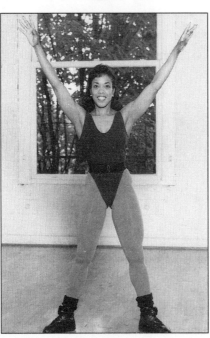
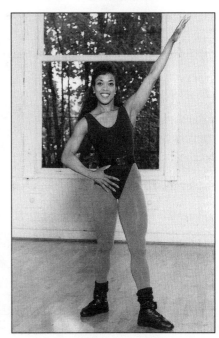

Sexy Walk

Four count, walking foward and crossing at ankles in relevé.

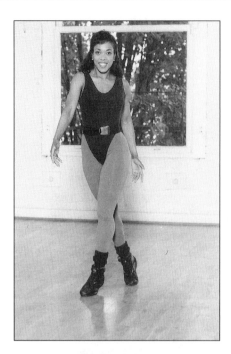
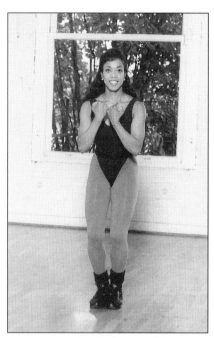

Swoop

1. Starting position: both feet together, hands at chest.

2. Left hip rotates out and left foot steps out laterally with arms sweeping down and then up.

3. Right foot steps over to bring both feet together, knees remain loose.

Repeat to right.

Cuing tip: left, close, right, close.

Total counts: 4

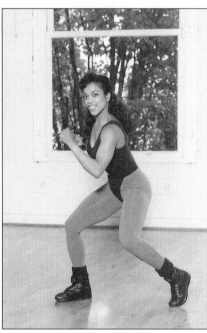
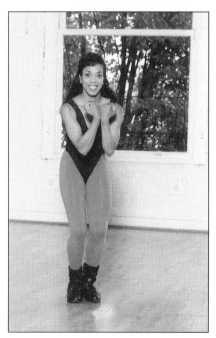

Run'n Man

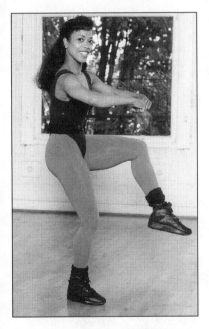 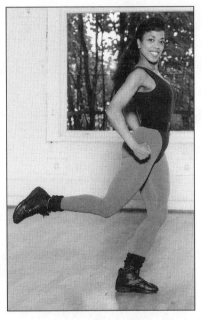 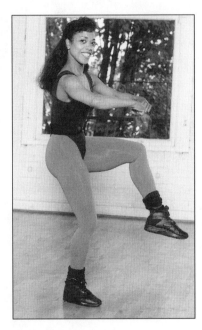

1. Right knee lifts. As you bring right leg back down, left leg slides back, all in one motion.

2. Left knee lifts. As you bring left leg back down, right leg slides back, all in one motion.

3. Repeat #1.

4. Repeat #2.

Cuing tip: knee, slide, knee, slide.

Total counts: 4

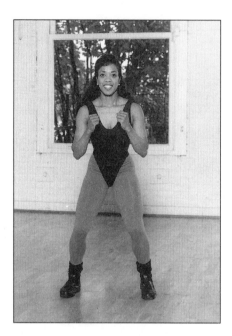
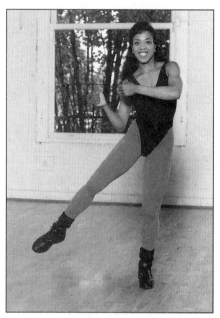

Troop

1. Stand with feet apart, knees bent, elbows tucked to waist, and hands clenched.

2. Brush floor with ball of left foot, lift left knee to side, lift shoulders, isolate ribs, both arms punch to left side.

3. Return to # 1.

4. Repeat #2, pressing off right side.

Total counts: 4

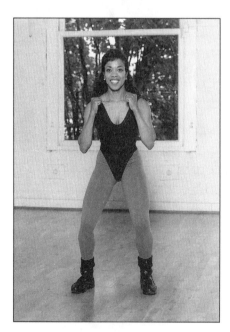
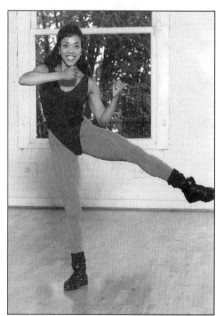

4 Taps with Hammer

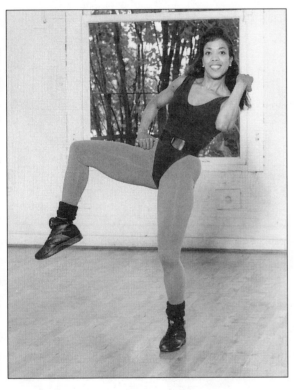

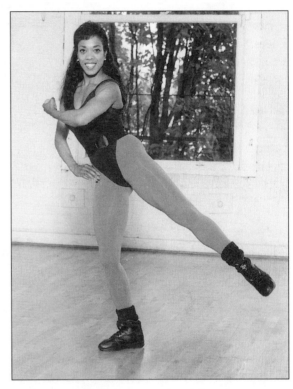

1. Upper body leans back with arm bent at elbow and hand in a fist pulled back by shoulder, with weight on supporting leg. Tap left foot.

2. As left foot goes down, shoulder lifts and hand comes down in front of abdominals, right leg extends behind body.

3. Repeat #1.

4. Repeat #2.

Cuing tip: travel four left, travel four right.

Total counts: 4

Roger Rabbit

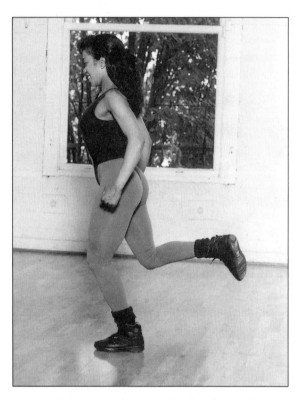 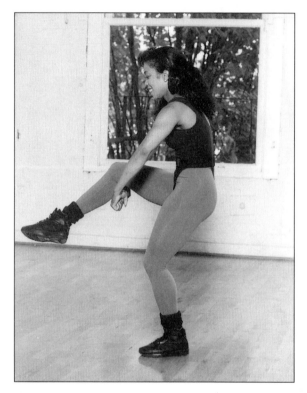

1. Step left, bring right leg back, elbows behind body, arching back.

2. Bring elbows forward, upper body curls forward, right knee lifts up.

3. Repeat #1 with right leg.

4. Repeat #2 and lift left knee.

Cuing tip: reverse skip.

Total counts: 4

Jazz Square

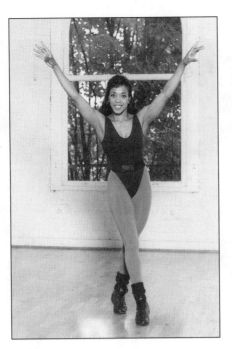
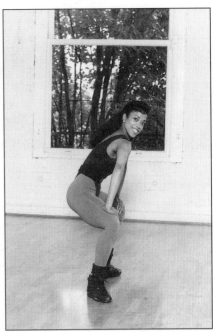

1. Left leg crosses over right ankle, arms in air in V position, lifting through center of body.

2. Right leg steps open to left side in ¼ turn, knees plié deep, back is flat, hands are placed on thighs.

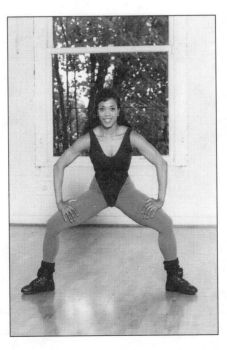
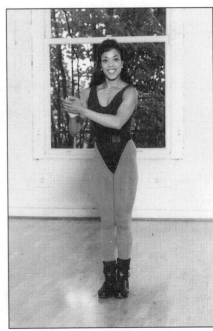

3. Remaining in plié position, lift left leg and ¼ turn to front.

4. Lift body to stand straight, bring right foot in to meet left foot, and clap.

Cuing tip: cross, open side, face front, step close.

Total counts: 4

Johnson Jamm

1. Second position plié, arms stacked, hands in fist.

2. Arms reverse and pull to opposite side, remaining in plié.

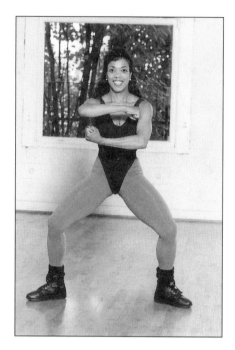
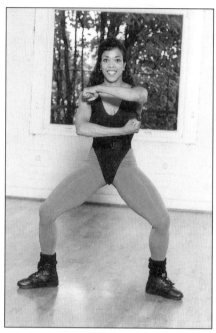

3. Both elbows come in to waist, palms up and lift hands to ceiling as if you were lifting a tray. Knees deep plié one count.

4. Repeat press up and deep plié one count.

Cuing tip: pull, pull, plié deep, plié deeper.

Total counts: 4

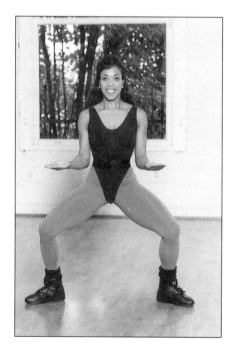
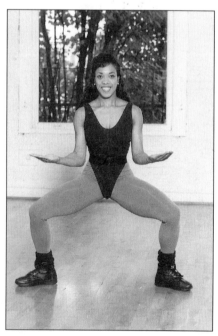

Stomp

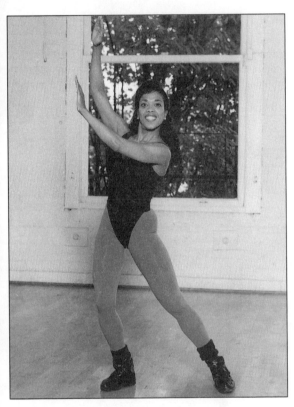

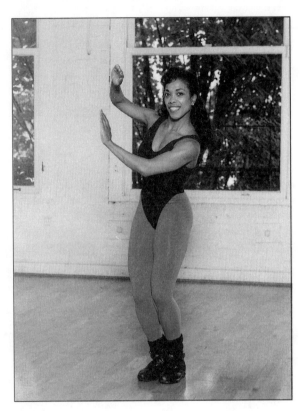

1. Step out to left, arms come above head in circular pattern (as if you were washing a window).

2. Step feet together, continue circular arm pattern.

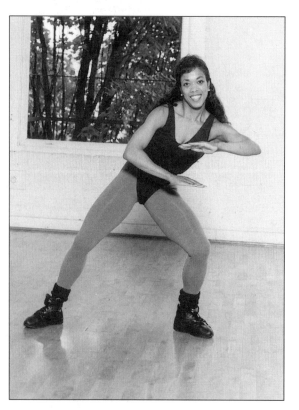

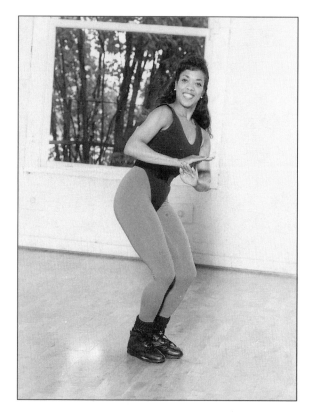

3. Step out and back to right, slight bend at waist and arms go in circular pattern below waist.

4. Step together and continue slight waist bend and washing pattern.

Cuing tip: step left, close, step right, close or wash up, wash down.

Total counts: 4

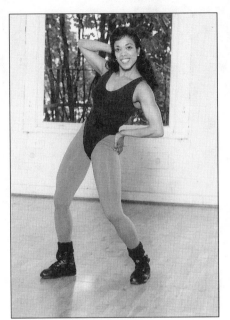
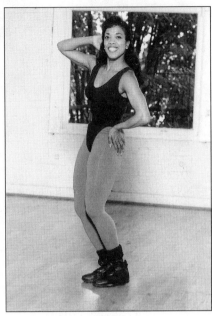

Sexy Stomp

Same as stomp with arm variation. One hand on hip, other behind head.

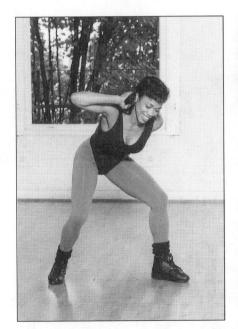
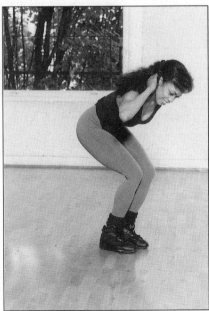

Chug

1. With arms bent at elbow and hands up by shoulders in a fist, press rib cage forward and pull shoulder blades together. Press shoulder back.

2. In one count, press elbows away and forward from body, rotate fists in to chest. Shoulders separate and lift, rib cage contracts. The motion will propel you in a small forward hop.

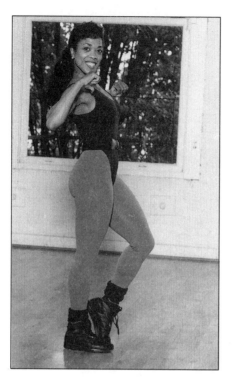
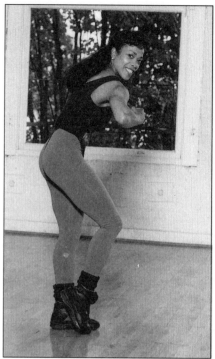

3. Repeat #1.

4. Repeat #2.

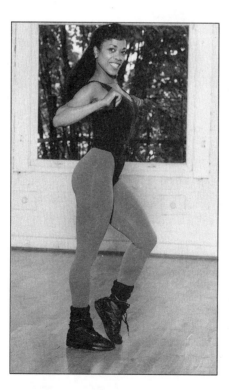
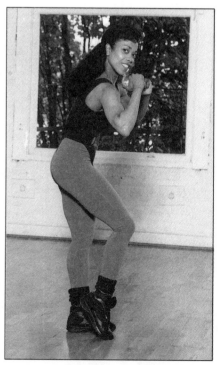

Vogue Chug

1. Left hand to head, right knee releases forward with a small hop.

2. Right hand to head, left knee releases forward with a small hop.

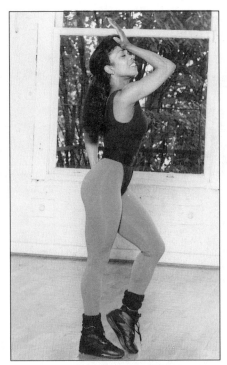 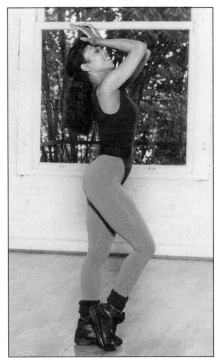

3. Both arms come down to waist with elbows bent, left knee releases forward with a small hop.

4. Both arms press down to side, right knee releases forward with a small hop.

Cuing tip: head, head, palms up, palms down.

Total counts: 4

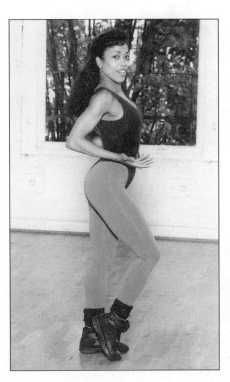 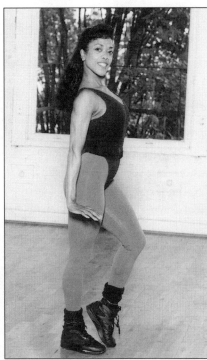

Fast Feet Pattern — Windmills

1. Feet together with knees slightly bent, arms bent at waist.

2. In one count, lift right arm above head, left arm crosses body, left leg opens out to side with heel down, toe lifted.

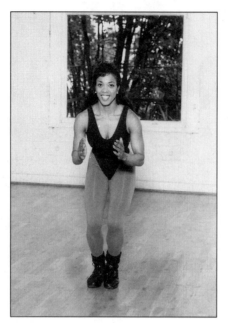
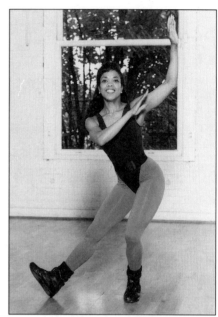

3. In one count return to #1.

4. In one count, lift left arm above head, right arm crosses body, right leg opens out to side with heel down, toe lifted.

Cuing tip: heel jack, close, heel jack, close.

Total counts: 4

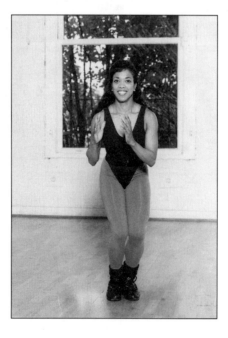
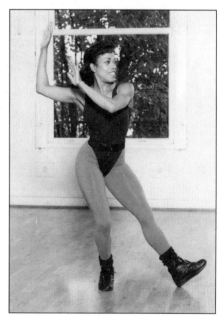

Funky Lunge

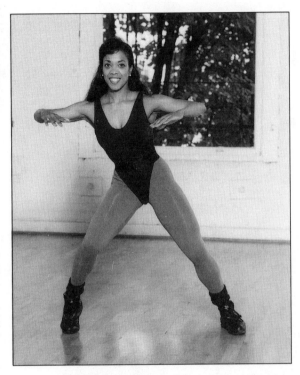 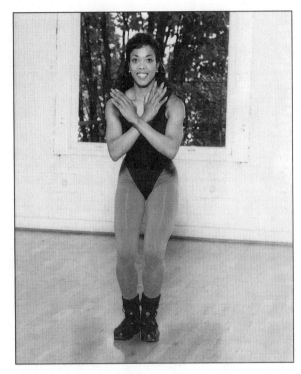

1. In one count, bring feet apart with weight on left leg, arms lift laterally.

2. Feet together with slight bend at waist, arms crossed over chest and knees soft.

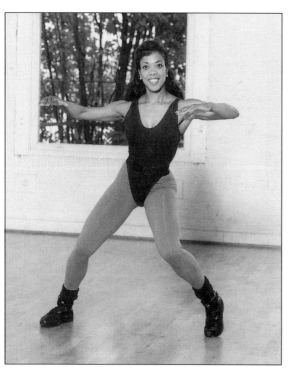

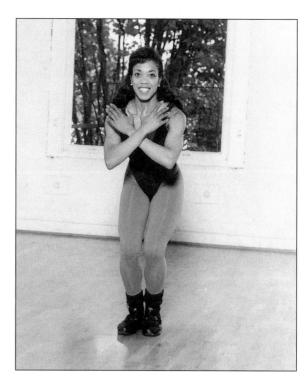

3. In one count, bring feet apart with weight on right leg, arms lift laterally.

4. Repeat #2.

Chapter Fifteen:
Technifunk™ Dance Workouts

Level 1 — Beginner

If you are new to working out, don't overload yourself with too much at one time. Get used to the new style of movement that you will be experiencing. Funk is totally different and unique, so be patient with yourself and your ability to perform each movement. If you are a beginner to exercise, work out along the following time line:

Warm-up preparation and stretch: 8 to 10 minutes
Technifunk™ Dance workout: 10 to 15 minutes
Cool-down and flexibility stretch: 8 to 10 minutes

Level 2 — Intermediate
Level 3 — Advanced

If you are familiar with aerobic exercise and dance training, this new movement may come a little easier and you will get an effective workout along the following time line:

Warm-up preparation and stretch: 8 to 10 minutes
Technifunk™ Dance workout: 20 to 40 minutes
Cool-down and flexibility stretch: 10 minutes

Beginner — Intermediate — Advanced Technifunk™ Dance Workout

(Total Minutes: 35 to 50)

Warm-up preparation and stretch: 8 to 10 minutes
Repeat each movement 8 to 16 times.
(See Chapter Six for movement descriptions.)

Deep Breathing
Pelvic Tilt
Pelvic Tilt with Spine Isolation
Shoulder Rotation
Shoulder Rolls
Torso Isolations

JAZZ ISOLATION SERIES

Rib-Cage Isolation
Hip Isolation
Chest Cross
Parallel Passé
Bicep Curl/Hip Isolation

STATIC ISOLATION STRETCH

Runner's Lunge
Calf Stretch
Hamstring Isolation
Groin Isolation
Posterior Shoulder Stretch
Anterior Shoulder Stretch
Head Tilt
Chin to Chest

TECHNIFUNK™ DANCE WORKOUT:

1. March — 1 minute
2. Wide step — 4 x
3. March — 16 counts
4. Wide step — 4 x
(Repeat 2 minutes)
5. Sexy Walk forward, 4 counts
6. Wide step — 2 x
7. Sexy Walk back, 4 counts
8. Wide step — 2 x
(Repeat sequence #5 to #8 approximately 3 minutes)
9. Swoop (in place, 2 minutes)
10. Swoop forward, 4 counts
11. Swoop in place, 4 counts
12. Swoop back, 4 counts
13. Swoop in place
(Repeat sequence #10 to #13 approximately 3 minutes)
Repeat combinations: #5 to #8 and #10 to #13 (2 minutes)
14. 4 Taps with Hammer to right

15. Run'n Man in place, 4 counts
16. 4 Taps with Hammer to left
17. Run'n Man in place, 4 counts
(Repeat sequence #14 to #17 approximately 2 minutes)
18. ¼ turn body to side and 4 Taps with Hammer traveling
    forward, ½ turn, repeat 4 Taps with Hammer traveling
    forward, 8 counts
19. Roger Rabbit back, 8 counts

(Repeat #18 to #19 approximately 2 minutes)
(This is the end of beginner workout; continue with cool-down.)

Intermediate and advanced — elapsed time: 15 minutes

Repeat combinations as follows:
#5 to #8
#10 to #13
#14 to #17
#18 to #19

20. Funky lunge 4 times
21. March in place 4 times
(Repeat #20 to #21 approximately 2 minutes)

22. Chug forward, 4 counts
23. Roger Rabbit back, 4 counts
24. Jazz Square
(Repeat #22 to #24 — 3 minutes)

Repeat combinations as follows:
(Advanced: Repeat 2 times)

#5 to #8
#10 to #13
#14 to #17
#18 to #19
#20 to #21
#22 to #24

Intermediate — **elapsed time: 26 minutes**
Advanced — **elapsed time: 29 minutes**

25. Johnson Jamm
26. Vogue Chug forward
27. Roger Rabbit back
28. Johnson Jamm
(Repeat sequence #25 to #28 — 4 minutes)
(This is the end of intermediate workout; continue with cool-down.)

29. Windmills
(Repeat, 1 minute)

Repeat sequence as follows:
 #5 to #8
#10 to #13
#14 to #17
#18 to #19
#20 to #21
#22 to #24
#25 to #28
#29
Repeat 2 times
Advanced — **elapsed time: 37 minutes**

COOL-DOWN:

Grapevine side to side — 1 minute
Chest Cross
Chest Press
Parallel Passé
Bicep Curl/Hip Isolation
Pullback
Calf Stretch
Hamstring Isolation #1
Groin Isolation #2

This is the end of your Technifunk™ Dance workout. Your options include moving on to specialty isolation stretches or going on to the Body Sculpting moves.

Final note: This workout does not include all the moves outlined in the Technifunk™ Dance section. As you become familiar with the workouts and you are ready to give Hammer a little competition, add the other movements to your jam session.

Afterword

I Choose

Our time together in this book is almost up, but our individual life-training journeys go on and on. Each of us is unique and has something very special to offer in this world. Starting right now I want you to break the cycle of self-doubt and self-destruction and work toward change. How can you give to others and begin making a difference in this life if you don't believe in yourself or take that first step toward changing the future? You can't pour from an empty cup, so every day strive to fill yours a little closer to the top.

Throughout this book I've just touched on the intricacies involved in subjects such as self-empowerment, motivation, self-esteem, and the importance of positive thinking and positive action. It may seem complex, and yet it all boils down to the same thing: choice. You choose who you are, you choose where you go, you choose what you do in life. Even when I was so physically and emotionally unhealthy, those were *my* choices. No one held me down, took a spoon, and shoveled food in my mouth. *I* picked up the spoon, and *I* swallowed — *all by myself.*

Being an educator at the forefront of fitness in this decade is an honor to me. To be an African-American female educator and serve as a role model is even more honorable. Traditionally, exercise has not been a part of my culture. However, today is a new day, and I believe it's time for African Americans (as well as other minorities in this country) to have the quality of life we all deserve. For this to happen will require that everyone get in the best physical and mental shape possible. Most kids I see play sports in hopes of landing an NBA contract, but the actual chances of that happening are next to none. Get fit and get an education first, and then work toward that NBA contract, if that is your goal. Learn to like and accept yourself.

My goal in writing this book was not simply to create another "workout book." My goal was to create a kind of "life training workbook" in which I offered tools and techniques for facing up to and conquering whatever challenges or opportunities life throws your way, as well as for improving the overall condition of your health and physical fitness. All of these things are encompassed in an *attitude* that I live by daily. My mission in life is to encourage other people to feel good about themselves and help them realize their own unique and special potential. Whenever you succeed at something, you create a "magic" that can become contagious—if you let it. Choose to believe in yourself and in your ability to succeed. There is great power in believing. Keep the faith and don't lose the magic. Never stop believing and keep your eyes on the prize. What's the prize? That's easy: The prize is whatever you want it to be—it's whatever you choose.

I Choose . . .

To live by choice, not by chance.
To make changes, not excuses.
To be motivated, not manipulated.
To be useful, not used.
To excel, not compete.

I choose self-esteem, not self-pity.
I choose to listen to the inner voice,
not the random opinions of others. . . .

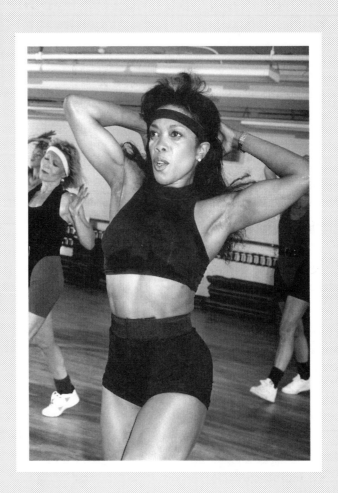

Videos by Victoria Johnson

TECHNIFUNK™ 2000
Instructor Dance Training
Funk Workout
90 minutes

Combines the freedom and innovation of funk with the disciplines of traditional dance technique. Jazz, ballet, modern dance, Hip-Hop, and traditional African dance are all combined to create a unique fitness experience. Designed for anyone who wants to dance for fitness, recreation, or performance. If you love to dance, Technifunk™ 2000 will move you into the outer limits of energy. Rated by *Self* and *American Health* magazines as best video of the year.
This video includes:

- State-of-the-art technique
- Breaks down over 20 of the hottest dance moves
- 45-minute workout of funk, fun, and excitement using combinations of all the moves
- Create your own routines and combinations

TECHNIFUNK™ II
The Dance Attack
30 minutes

This all-out dance workout combines jazz, ballet, and Hip-Hop funk movements for an energy-filled DANCE ATTACK! Not only will you burn fat and shape up, you will be movin' your body in ways you never imagined possible! This is your chance to enjoy the freedom of movement and experience the infectious energy and motivation that Victoria has brought to the world of fitness!
Technifunk™ II, The Dance Attack
- 30 minutes of pure energy
- Easy to follow
- Motivational workout
- Funky dance moves
- Burns fat!

DANCE STEP FORMULA
Latest Step Workout
70 minutes

Dance Step Formula is the fusion of funky dance and step choreography. Excellent fat-burning workout plus great sculpting for the hips, buns, and thighs. Victoria is pumpin' up the jam with her own unique combination of STEP & TECHNIFUNK™! "It is time for a more balanced program," says Victoria. "This video will give you that while utilizing dance technique to enhance the step workout."
- Unique transitions from dance to step
- Funk grooves and Hip-Hop moves
- Challenging funk and step combinations
- Powerful body shaping with step strap
- 60 minutes of pure excitement

STEP AND SHAPE
Basic/intermediate step training
30 minutes

Step training is easy to learn, yet it's the most advanced form of exercise possible. Results are fast and noticeable in the hips, buns, thighs, and upper body. Stepping is one of the best aerobic workouts, building stamina and increasing endurance while it's easy on the knees and ankles. Burn fat and firm up every major muscle group. Victoria's sizzling dance tracks and unbeatable attitude will have you smiling from the first step to the last!

H.A.B.I.T.
Hips, Abs, Buns, Incredible Thighs
30 minutes

Zero in on those trouble spots: buttocks, hips, stomach, and upper thighs. Combining floor work and sophisticated vertical exercises, Victoria has developed a 30 minute program that gets results quickly. Lose inches fast! Add hand weights when you're ready. Special emphasis on abdominals! Terrific dance tracks and Victoria's non-stop enthusiasm will keep you going from beginning to end!

TOTAL BODY WORKOUT
Aerobics — basic/intermediate
30 minutes

With a sizzling sound track, a solid high-energy, low-impact power workout, and Victoria's pump-it-up attitude, you'll be revved up from top to bottom! Burn fat while trimming and shaping every part of your body. Light hand weights come into play during the body-shaping segment. A great "multi-level" workout — designed so that anyone can do it.

CARDIO POWER CROSSTRAINING WORKOUT
Crosstraining — Aerobic/Toning/Funk/Floor work
65 minutes

Victoria's Cardio Power Crosstraining Workout gives you a total body workout in just 60 minutes. Divided into five segments, the program allows you to choose one or all exercise groups for a customized, focused workout. Whatever you choose, these workouts guarantee increased endurance and energy, improve muscle tone, and lower overall body fat. The Total Fitness Program is a high-tech, multi-fitness experience. Components of this crosstraining workout include:

- Rhythmic dance warm-up
- High-energy cardio patterns
- Cardio-power weight training
- Funk kool-down
- Toning, shaping floor work

For more information write or call:
Metro Fitness
Box 1744
Lake Oswego, OR 97035
1-800-635-3893